Ti... Without Surgery

"Too often surgery is considered early on in the treatment process for back pain. This refreshing book provides insight into the many non-surgical alternatives that could and should be explored in conjunction with competent medical authority prior to surgical intervention. These alternatives, in many instances, would be consistent with the approach desired from the business community which seeks appropriate, cost-effective quality outcomes. Ultimately, it will be the patient who is best served through non-surgical alternatives advanced by this book!"

—Joseph B. Freeman, Jr., Executive Director, Savannah Business Group on Health Care Cost Management

"*Treat Your Back Without Surgery* will empower the back or neck pain sufferer to play an active role in the prevention and treatment of their disease. The instructions in early non-surgical intervention will delay or eliminate the need for surgery."

— Pam Thomas, M.D., Medical Director, Lockheed Martin

"With millions of people suffering from back pain every day, it's extremely important that all available options be reviewed. While surgery is one option, this book provides a great overview of many non-surgical alternatives that are equally effective."

— Cheryl Tanigawa, M.D., Medical Director, PacifiCare of California

"Large employers want the best value health care for their employees. *Treat Your Back Without Surgery* gives the reader an overview of the non-surgical treatment alternatives to be explored by the back pain sufferer before resorting to surgery. This information would be valuable to anyone suffering from back pain who is searching for an effective route back to activity."

— Sue Nelson, Worldwide Director,
Health Benefits & Services, Texas Instruments

"In my 38 years of rehabilitation and sports medicine practice, approximately 85% of the post-surgical rehab patients we have treated would not have needed surgery if they would have been able to read this book. It offers a comprehensive knowledge of the alternatives to immediate surgery, and addresses the need for people to learn how to enter the therapeutic process that will help them care for their own backs. Readers can develop a safe, preventative, and even corrective approach to acute and chronic back pain prior to needing surgery."

— Wayne R. English, Jr. D.O., Texas College of Osteopathic Medicine

Dedication

This book is dedicated to all back pain sufferers with a hope that properly applied knowledge might alleviate or prevent future back discomfort.

— Stephen Hochschuler, M.D.

To my wife Wendy and our three sons John, Mark, and Andrew, whose patience and understanding during many months of research and writing made this book possible.

— Bob Reznik

Treat Your Back Without Surgery

The best non-surgical alternatives for eliminating back and neck pain

Stephen Hochschuler, M.D.
&
Bob Reznik, MBA

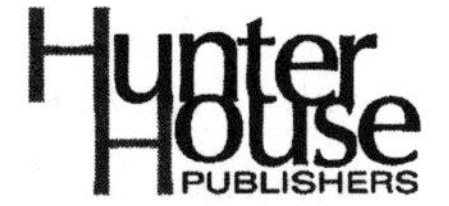

Hunter House Inc., Publishers
P.O. Box 2914, Alameda, CA 94501-0914

Exercise Photos: Paul Buck
Model: Shannon Hanlon, Personal Trainer, Southlake Training Center

Library of Congress Cataloging-in-Publication Data
Hochschuler, Stephen.
Treat your back without surgery : an educated consumer's guide to the best non-surgical alternatives for eliminating back and neck pain / Stephen Hochschuler, Bob Reznik.
p. cm.
Includes bibliographical references and index.
ISBN 0-89793-234-X (alk. paper). — ISBN 0-89793-235-8 (cloth)
1. Backache—Prevention. 2. Backache—Treatment. 3. Back—Care and hygiene. 4. Backache—Exercise therapy. 5. Self-care, Health. I. Reznik, Bob. II. Title.
RD771.B217H645 1998
617.5'64—dc21 98-4613
CIP

Ordering
Hunter House books are available at bulk discounts for textbook course adoptions, to qualifying community, healthcare, and government organizations, and for special promotions and fundraising. For details please contact:

Special Sales Department
Hunter House Inc., PO Box 2914, Alameda CA 94501-0914
Tel. (510) 865-5282 Fax (510) 865-4295
e-mail: marketing@hunterhouse.com

Individuals can order our books from most bookstores or by calling toll-free:
1-800-266-5592

Cover Design: Jil Weil Graphic Design
Book Design: Cameron Dobson, Prizm Development, Inc.
Project Coordinators: Wendy Low, Belinda Breyer
Editors: Belinda Breyer, Kevin Bentley, Kiran S. Rana Indexer: ALTA Indexing
Marketing: Corrine M. Sahli Special Sales: Susan Markey
Customer Support: Christina Arciniega and Edgar M. Estavilla, Jr.
Publisher: Kiran S. Rana

Printed and Bound by Publishers Press, Salt Lake City, UT
Manufactured in the United States of America

9 8 7 6 5 4 3 2 1 First Edition

Contents

A notice about the risks you assume with self-care

In this book we have tried to present a review of helpful information regarding back care without the confusing jargon found in medical textbooks. The contents are based on current information, professional research, and consultation with other medical professionals. Every effort has been made to provide accurate, dependable, and up-to-date information, including an overview of alternative and some unproven therapies.

With that said, this book is *not* intended to replace the doctor-patient relationship. No book can replace the care and judgment of a physician or a spine specialist, or make you an expert in medical diagnosis. Instead, this book is intended to help you understand more about your back or neck problem so that when you visit your physician, you will be better informed and able to discuss your problem. The treatments described in the book should be undertaken only under the guidance of a licensed healthcare practitioner. Self-care and home remedies that may be appropriate for one person may be inappropriate for another — your doctor is the best person to decide after evaluating your specific case. Generally speaking, when self-care does not relieve symptoms over a couple days, you should seek the help of a doctor.

The reader is warned that those people who diagnose and treat themselves do so at their own risk. The authors and the publisher assume no responsibility for any problems that may result from using the information provided in this book in a program of self-care or under the care of a licensed practitioner. Finally, as advances in medical and scientific research are made very quickly, the authors, publisher, editors, and professionals quoted in the book cannot be held responsible for any error, omission, or dated material.

Authors' Preface

The trend in medicine today is to explore nonsurgical solutions to various health problems. For example, Dr. Dean Ornish's book, *Dr. Dean Ornish's Program for Reversing Heart Disease,* has become a best seller among consumers and doctors. His nonsurgical treatment regimen, which at the time raised a lot of eyebrows in the medical community, is now endorsed by many cardiologists as an alternative to heart bypass surgery. Dr. Ornish has shown that, through changes in diet and exercise, many people who previously would have undergone heart surgery can now reverse their heart disease without surgery.

Now, this same trend is occurring in the area of spine care, providing a fresh approach to treating and relieving back and neck pain.

We believe consumers are the driving force in the effort to improve quality in the health care industry. Unlike their parents, who often blindly followed the recommendations of physicians, middle-aged baby boomers are asking questions, researching their own health care problems, surfing health care Internet sites, and putting their doctors on the spot.

Back pain sufferers in the United States have far more back and neck surgery than those in other countries. Worse, the outcome from spine surgery can be disastrous when performed by surgeons who do not perform a high volume of back surgery and are not proficient in the techniques. This book provides an overview of the many nonsurgical alternatives available to relieve back and neck pain, in the belief that in more than 95 percent of cases, surgery should be held out as the last and most final option.

Acknowledgments

The authors received the input of several experts around the country to make this book more balanced in its presentation. For their contributions to chapters mentioned, the authors extend thanks:

Chapters 2 & 3

Matt Michaels, M.D., specialist in Physical Medicine & Rehabilitation and Medical Director of Tennessee Spine, Memphis, Tennessee.

Chapters 3 & 4

Steve Winkler, Director of Rehabilitation, Center for Spine, Savannah, Georgia; John Triano, D.C., Director of Chiropractic at the Texas Back Institute.

Chapter 6

Wayne R. English, Jr., D.O., Clinical Professor, University of North Texas Health Science Center/Texas College of Osteopathic Medicine, Fort Worth, Texas. Dr. English is a specialist in Physical Medicine and Rehabilitation. Also, Steven M. Taylor, D.O., Director of Research, Center for Pain Management, Fort Worth, Texas. Dr. Taylor is board-certified in Pain Management.

Chapter 11

Lawrence Miller, M.D., Coast Pain Management, Fountain Valley, California. Dr. Miller is board-certified in internal medicine, anesthesiology and pain management. Also contributing from Coast Pain Management were Michael Lowenstein, M.D. and Clifford Bernstein, M.D., both board-certified in pain management and anesthesiology. Also, Ralph Rashbaum, M.D., co-founder and medical director, the Texas Back Institute.

PART 1

Understanding Back and Neck Pain

CHAPTER 1

How You Can Benefit from This Book

You are probably reading this page right now because you have back or neck pain. Or it may be that your husband, wife, child, Mom, or Dad has back pain and you are the one who is trying to sort out what to do about it. If you are a back or neck pain sufferer yourself, you are probably afraid of what the future may hold for you. Are you going to be paralyzed? Are you going to end up in a wheelchair? Is there something seriously wrong in your back that may require a surgery? Will you ever be able to play your favorite sport or enjoy your favorite activity again? Or will you even be able to go back to work and make a living?

Back and neck pain can cause these and other fears and doubts to race through your mind. The fear of the unknown can stop you from doing anything physical in case you hurt yourself even more, so you do less and less. This lack of activity in turn causes muscles and tendons in your back to become weaker and less flexible, so they are susceptible to strain from simple things, like bending over to pick up your child or adjust the TV set. The less you do, the more simple things hurt, a vicious cycle that can drag you down into a disability spiral.

The unknowns are particularly difficult to cope with when suffering from back or neck pain. So here are some "knowns" that you may find immediately comforting.

The "80 percent" rule for back and neck pain

1. Eighty percent of Americans will have back or neck pain at some time in their lives.
2. Eighty percent of back and neck pain is muscle related.
3. Eighty percent of back and neck pain will go away on its own over time with a little help from Mother Nature.

There are a lot of people hurting, so you are not alone. For most of us, the pain is temporary, not permanently damaging to the spine, and will go away on its own.

But how do you get from where you are now back to activity? And what if you are not among that lucky 80 percent? What if you are one of that horrible 20 percent, whose back or neck pain is more serious than just muscle strain? What if you are among that 20 percent of people whose back or neck pain has *not* gone away on its own?

This book is for both groups: the 80 percent *and* the 20 percent. It will help you learn what may be causing your back or neck pain, and what to do about it. As such, you will learn about a wide variety of potential cures and treatments for your back pain, many of which you may never have heard of before. Some may sound unusual. Some are cures people in other countries use successfully to recover from back pain. We have tried to provide an overview of many types of non-surgical cures for back and neck pain — with comment but without too much judgment. Our premise is that virtually any non-surgical treatment that will not make you worse may be worth a try before you resort to surgery.

The small number of people with back pain who may actually need back or neck surgery will also benefit from this book because they will learn how to select a surgeon, how to make sure they are getting the right type of surgery, and the right rehabilitation procedures to follow after surgery.

Pain relief, then prevention

Our hope is that this book could be a godsend for those people who have had back or neck pain for some time and have struggled to find a long-lasting solution, or are relying on medication, or are considering surgery as a permanent solution.

Our first goal is to help you get past your current pain symptoms, our second goal is to help you to prevent your next back pain attack.

Let's assume we can provide a non-surgical alternative treatment for you that relieves your pain. To prevent that back problem from returning tomorrow, you must change the musculature in your spine. You must make your back stronger, more flexible, and injury resistant.

In this book you will learn specific exercises that can strengthen your back or neck and make it more flexible and injury resistant. Knowing the right way to lift, push, or pull can also eliminate the common motions that cause a back strain. Just as you alter your diet to improve your cholesterol level, you *can* take action to lower your risk of back pain in the future. We will show you how.

Through this book, you will learn that surgery isn't the cure to explore *first*, as some doctors may lead you to believe. Surgery is the cure to explore *last*. We'll tell you why, and reveal the kinds of complications that most people don't learn about until it's too late and they have reached a point of no return.

Can my back pain go away with exercise?

About 90 percent of back pain sufferers get better within a couple of months. Unfortunately, studies estimate that, at any given time, about 8 percent of Americans suffer from chronic pain, of which a large part is back pain. The bad news is that for those whose back pain does not go away over the first six months, it may stick around off and on for years. Liberty Mutual has noted in research about disability that the longer a person is off work because of back pain, the lower the chance of them ever returning to work. Only 50 percent of those off work for six months from a back injury return to work. After two years of disability, the odds of someone returning to work are virtually nil.

Worse, once a person falls into the chronic pain abyss, they sometimes fall victim to other health problems. Some researchers observe that 75 percent of chronic pain sufferers complain about multiple health problems.

Who is at high risk for a back attack?

Is there any way to tell if you are a back attack waiting to happen? If you are middle-aged and work, you have a bull's-eye on your back. That's because back pain is a middle-aged, working person's problem. It cuts across all demographic and occupational groups, from college professors to nurses to garbage collectors. The age when most of us are at risk for back pain is between 35 and 55 — prime working age. Men and women are at equal risk for lower back pain, and in women there is some indication that there is increased prevalence of lower back pain after menopause.

While men and women suffer from back pain equally, research done by Prizm Development, Inc., in the United States shows that 60 percent of people who seek help for back pain are female. Women don't have more back pain than men, it is just that they are more likely to go to the doctor for their problem, while men may put off going to the doctor out of fear.

Researchers note that physical fitness is not a predictor of risk for lower back pain, but they do note that if a person is physically fit they are likely to recover more quickly after a pain episode.

What you will learn from this book

In this book, you will learn that even before you have an MRI or other diagnostic test, you can know your odds of having a herniated disc.

You will learn that if you live in the southern United States, the likelihood of your having back surgery is significantly higher than if you live in California.

You will learn the best treatment for various back and neck problems, even though this may be different from the treatment you are currently getting from your doctor.

You will learn that, compared with the United States, other countries use surgery half as frequently to treat back or neck pain.

You will learn alternative methods of back care that will get you active again without surgery. These include mainstream treatments that are widely accepted by the best spine centers in the world. This book also covers non-traditional methods that may help you relieve back and neck pain — all without surgery.

You will learn how to evaluate and treat your back pain with home remedies and a customized exercise program that you can do in your home, in the gym, at work, or on the golf course.

You will learn what symptoms indicate the need for professional help, and how to search for a spine physician who will give you the care you need to treat your back without surgery. If you really do need surgery, you will learn how to find the kind of surgeon who can increase your odds of a successful surgical outcome. You can even check their credentials in advance on the Internet.

Lastly, the most important thing you will learn from this book is that there is really only one person you can trust with your welfare — you. When it comes to back or neck pain, especially back or neck surgery, you must quickly become an educated consumer. You cannot abdicate responsibility for your health to someone else. You must play an active role in your care and in your recovery.

Who you select as your back or neck doctor will have a tremendous impact on the rest of your life. You must find a doctor who is open to all the possible non-surgical treatment alternatives available for back or neck pain.

Becoming informed

As with any other professional service, if you don't become an educated consumer when seeking back and neck pain treatment, you may get ripped off. Only in this case it's "ripped open." Some spine physicians estimate that half the back and neck surgeries that are performed in the United States may be unnecessary.

Making the wrong decision about back treatment is not like making a bad decision on a new car purchase — you can't exchange your back if you make the wrong choice. You could be stuck with a bad back for life. It is truly amazing how people will immerse themselves in researching the purchase of a new car, VCR, or big-screen television, yet they will trust their spine care to anyone in a white coat.

Back and neck pain, like chest pain, is a signal from your body to your brain that something is wrong. We all know that chest pain is not something you ignore. Chest pain could mean a heart attack, and that could be fatal. While a "back attack" won't be fatal to your life, it could be fatal to your lifestyle. Instead of a full and active life, you may be couch-bound.

The authors' perspectives

Together, the authors have played key roles in developing the nation's largest spine center of excellence — the Texas Back Institute. In 1995, 10,000 spine patients traveled to the Texas Back Institute. One in five had previously had spine surgery performed by other doctors that didn't work. Many patients, in fact, had *multiple* spine surgeries elsewhere. For example, one patient had 24 back surgeries before coming to the Texas Back Institute.

Texas Back Institute physicians have seen tragedies up close. Tragedies because, in some cases, patients should never have had a first surgery, let alone a second.

Unlike other books on back pain, often written by an expert with an inherent treatment bias, this book has a balanced and healthy perspective on back and neck pain.

The first perspective is that of a spine surgeon who has performed several thousand spine surgeries during a career at the Texas

Back Institute, and has helped tens of thousands find relief *without* surgery. Interestingly, as a long-term back pain sufferer himself, Dr. Hochschuler has never given in to surgery. Every back attack has been defended against with a dedication to non-surgical cures and the belief that over time, with perseverance, the symptoms will go away. Perhaps you too can find non-surgical relief with the medical information Dr. Hochschuler provides in this book.

The second perspective we offer is that of a consumer advocate. Bob Reznik holds a master's degree in business administration with specialization in the area of healthcare management and quality systems. Reznik, as president of Prizm Development, Inc., helps quality-minded physician groups improve the way they take care of patients. Prizm believes strongly that to get the best quality out of the health care system, the consumer must be educated and well-informed. Prizm, in the course of its business, has had extensive meetings with more than one hundred HMO medical directors and the employee benefit managers at large companies from across the United States. You will learn how these large purchasers, who are shopping for quality, look at the field of spine care. Coincidentally, most managed care organizations and large companies are demanding a non-surgical approach to back and neck pain.

Thirdly, this book has been intentionally balanced with the input of specialists in pain management, physical medicine, and physical therapy, from the East Coast to the West Coast, who have contributed their insights to various chapters that relate to their area of expertise.

Not surprisingly, all involved believe that finding high quality in healthcare starts with the consumer. You must search for the right doctor, and then play an active role in your treatment and recovery. You must ask questions at every turn.

Through this book, you will learn the questions to ask.

Through this book we hope to help you understand what may be causing your back or neck pain, and how to find relief from it without surgery.

CHAPTER 2

How Your Back Works and What Can Go Wrong With It

Let's say you have just had an MRI (magnetic resonance imaging) scan at the doctor's office and now you are waiting for the results. Let me be the first to break the bad news to you.

Hang onto your hat. It's pretty safe to say that you have a herniated disc, or at least a bulging disc, in your spine. How do we know that, not having seen you? Let's just say we have some inside information.

In fact, if you are over 60, we'll bet you hands down that you have an "abnormal MRI." We can make that bet with the calculated assurance of a Las Vegas MBA who re-sets the odds on the slot machines in the casino lobby every Sunday before the vacationers leave for the airport.

In a study published in the *Journal of Bone & Joint Surgery*, researchers performed MRI scans on 67 healthy people who had never had back pain. The scans were then interpreted independently by three different neuro-radiologists, the best possible specialists to read MRI scans. None of the three radiologists had any knowledge of the absence or presence of back pain symptoms in the scanned patients.

The results? One-third of all the healthy people were diagnosed with a spine abnormality like a herniated disc. Of those under age 60, 20 percent had a herniated disc. Of those over 60, 57 percent had a spine abnormality, 36 percent had a herniated disc, and 21 percent had stenosis, a narrowing of the spinal canal. Even in the youngest group of healthy patients, those 20 to 39 years old, 35% had a degenerating or bulging disc. And of those over 60, all but one subject had a degenerating or bulging disc.[1]

The researchers found that before a surgeon comes to the conclusion that a person's back pain is caused by the disc abnormality that shows up on a MRI scan, they should consider that, as we get older, more and more of us look abnormal on film. Just as a camera catches all of our outside imperfections, it's fair to guess that nobody looks perfect on the inside either. All of which underscores the need to consider a non-surgical approach before giving up and opting for surgery.

Remember, a lot of healthy people have herniated discs. Because you have back pain and a herniated disc, that does not necessarily mean you need surgery.

For over 20 years, CT (computerized tomography) and MRI scans have provided physicians the technology to look inside our bodies and, as one would expect, it's not always a pretty picture. When a patient complains of back or neck pain, and an MRI scan reveals a herniated disc in that area, it is logical to associate one with the other.

From 1979 to 1990, the period that CT and MRI became commonplace in most cities, the rate of back surgery increased 55 percent, rising from 1.02 back surgeries per thousand people to 1.58 per thousand. The greatest increase was for spinal stenosis surgery, which more than quadrupled.[2]

Some physicians will give a back or neck pain sufferer drugs to mask the pain, and a sheet of paper with home exercises to follow as their physical therapy program. Guess how many people fail this non-surgical treatment program? With such a half-hearted effort at non-surgical resolution, it's not surprising that a lot of people never get better, and are moved along by the surgeon into the operating room.

Understanding how your spine works

To learn how to treat your back without surgery, you first need a little overview on how your spine is built, and which things can go wrong. After reviewing that we will show you how to fix the things that may be wrong. You will also need this information so you can communicate better with your doctor.

Throughout this book, we will use the word "back" to refer to the entire length of the spine, from the lower "lumbar" area all the way up to the "cervical" neck area. That's because the neck and lower back share the same anatomical parts, and both neck and lower back pain can come from muscle strain, disc problems, stenosis, traumatic injury, and arthritis.

The biggest difference may be how the lumbar and cervical areas become injured. The lumbar spine often becomes injured from lifting, pushing, or pulling. Neck strain comes from office work, such as sitting at a computer for long periods. Because neck muscles have to support the weight of the head, and holding a static position can be hard work, neck muscles can become strained. That's why office workers should always get up, move around, and do neck exercises that relax the neck muscles. More about that later in the book.

Both the neck and lower back can be injured by a fall or car accident. In fact, car accidents are more likely to hurt the neck than the lower back. In whiplash, the weight of the head moves forward and then snaps back, causing great strain on the neck.

Treatment of lumbar and neck strain focuses on strengthening the supporting muscles and tendons. Treating lumbar disc problems may focus on stabilizing the lower back, which has more lifting duty.

Spine overview The spine is really a complex tower of bones, discs, joints, muscles, and ligaments. The spinal column is composed of 25 bones, each called a vertebra (the plural is vertebrae), which are separated by shock-absorbing discs.

Protruding from the back side of each rounded vertebra body are the remaining components that make up the "posterior elements": the bony pedicles and laminae, the facet joints, and the bony transverse and spinous processes, which are the narrow, finger-like spikes pointing out from the sides and back of the vertebra.

This tower is held in place by surrounding muscles, ligaments, and tendons that act as supporting guy wires. When working properly, the spine is able bend and twist, thanks to hinge-like structures called facet joints and the flexibility of the discs.

Threaded through the protective vertebral bodies of the tower within the spinal canal is the body's internal electrical system, a bundle of nerves called the spinal cord.

To communicate with your back doctor, you'll need to learn the vocabulary. Your doctor may use terms like C-7, L-4, T-8. These terms relate to a numbering system on the spine tower.

Starting at the top at your head and working down your back, the spinal column is divided into three sections. Cervical vertebrae, designated C-1 through C-7, make up your neck area, and are smaller and

Spine Diagram

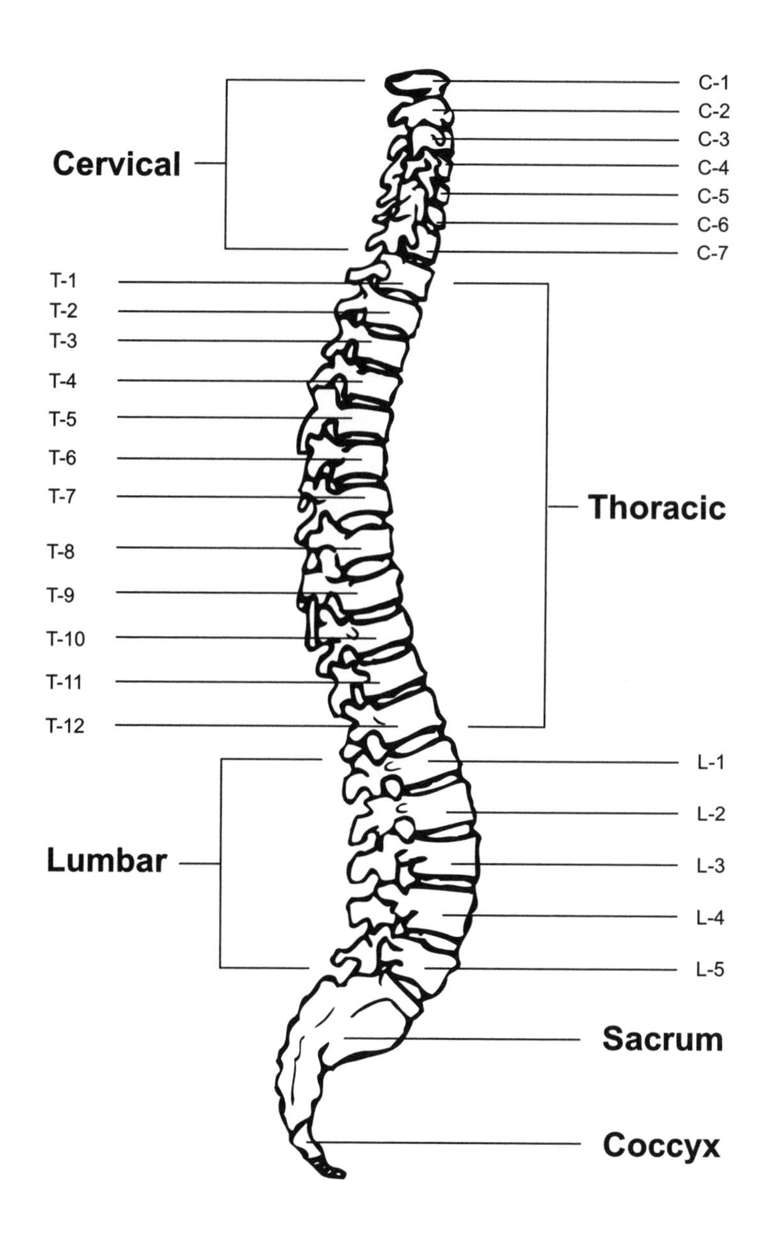

more fragile than those in the trunk. They also protect the portion of the spinal cord that attaches to the brain.

The chest area contains the thoracic vertebrae, T-1 through T-12. The thoracic vertebrae don't rotate as much as the neck and lower back. Consequently, this area of the spine is more stable and is generally less susceptible to injury. Relatively few back pain cases involve the T-level vertebrae.

The lumbar area, or lower back, contains L-1 through L-5, the largest, sturdiest group of vertebrae. But because it bears most of the body's weight as we sit, stand, push, pull, lift, and move, the lumbar section is considered the most injury-prone area of the spine.

The spinal cord threads from the brain down through the spine and ends at about L-2, after which it forms a bundle of nerves known as the *cauda equina* (Latin for "horse's tail"). From the neck area to the coccyx are 31 pairs of nerve roots that exit the spinal canal and head for remote areas of the body through vertebral portals called foramina.

At the base of L-5 is a solid mass of five fused bones called the sacrum (pronounced "say-crum"). Finally, the spinal column ends at the coccyx (pronounced "cock-six"), or tailbone. We count the sacrum and coccyx as one bone in the spine diagram because actually several small bones are fused together.

A healthy spine is slightly S-shaped when viewed from the side. From the front or back, though, the normal spine appears straight.

Understanding how your back muscles work

All over the back is a complex, intertwined network of muscles and ligaments that travel up and down the spine, and then spread sideways across the shoulders and lower back area. Because humans walk upright rather than on all fours, we have developed musculature that keeps the trunk stable while walking, running, bending, or lifting.

The many individual muscles and ligaments involving the trunk have enough Latin names to fill an entire chapter, or even a book. We'll just cover the key muscles here to give you a solid understanding of muscle anatomy and, more importantly, how these muscle groups work together.

The easiest way to understand back musculature is to think of the back as having three rubber bands that work together to keep the spine stable and in a neutral position. There is a big rubber band on the back that enables us to straighten, a big rubber band on the front that pulls us forward into a bending position, and a rubber band that wraps around our sides that helps keep everything stable. A problem with any one of the rubber bands can result in back pain. Rehabilitation from back strain, for example, typically involves a strengthening all three rubber bands, and making them all more flexible.

The rubber band analogy is especially appropriate because, just as rubber bands become dry, brittle, and prone to tearing as they get old, so do our back muscles. Also, the best way to keep a rubber band flexible and working well is to constantly stretch it, but not so far that it tears.

The musculature of the back can be grouped as follows:

Muscle Diagram

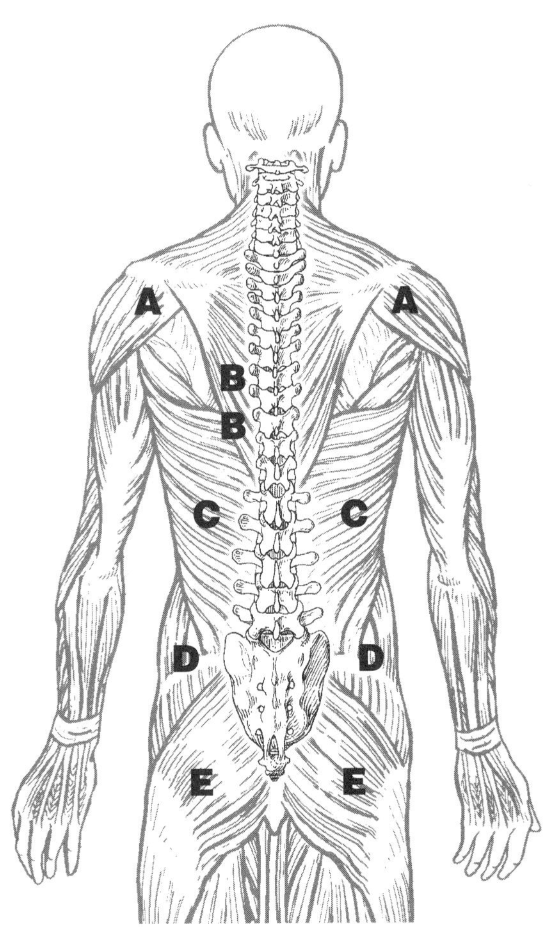

A *Rear deltoid muscles*
B *Trapezius muscles*
C *Latissimus dorsi muscles*
D *Oblique muscles*
E *Gluteal muscles, including the piriformis*

- Extensors — the muscles and tendons in our back that enable us to "extend" or arch backward. Any time you bend backward, stand, or straighten up from a sitting position, or perform lifting motions, you are using your extensor muscles.

- Flexors — the muscles in front that enable us to raise up from a prone position, as in doing a sit-up.

- Obliques — the muscles that travel around our sides that help balance and stabilize the trunk.

The extensor muscles, while they act like one big rubber band, are really a series of long and short muscles that travel up and down the back. When one of these muscles is strained, the resulting spasm may be excruciating.

The flexor muscles, also called the abdominals, are really your stomach muscles. They also assist in lifting. The abdominals work with the buttock muscles to support the spine.

The oblique muscles provide additional support to the spine and control the pelvis. Strong obliques can greatly reduce stress on the spine.

The large thigh muscles, called quadriceps, rarely strain but they play a supporting role in helping the back to lift. So in a rehab program your therapist may want you to strengthen these muscles to take the load off your back.

There are many specific muscles and muscle groups that play supporting roles. The latissimus dorsi muscles, for instance, (see figure on p. 18) stabilize the pelvic area. The buttock muscles, called gluteals, travel from the lower back area and attach to the legs.

The piriformis muscle lies under the buttock muscles and travels from the sacrum area (central lower back area) to the top of the leg. It helps with leg and hip movement, and can play a key role in lower back pain.

What makes this muscle especially important is that the sciatic nerve travels through it. Consequently, when the piriformis muscle tightens with strain or spasm it can affect the sciatic nerve, causing further pain into the leg.

Pain that radiates into the leg is also often associated with a herniated disc. In that case you have similar symptoms, but requiring radically different types of treatment. A disc problem may require surgery, but muscle strain does not.

This underscores the importance of having an experienced spine physician who can get to the bottom of the problem, so to speak.

What causes back and neck pain

Muscle strain This is a catch-all category, also called "soft tissue injury," which covers muscles, tendons, and ligaments. About 80% of back and neck pain is muscle-related. Surgery is never appropriate for muscle strain. A symptom of muscle strain may be an excruciating spasm in the back that makes you drop to your knees in pain.

Some people believe that part of what makes the back muscles more prone to strain is that they are shorter than other big muscles in the body. The muscles in our thighs that enable us to walk, run, and jump are longer and less prone to strain. It is very unusual to strain a thigh muscle.

Another type of strain relates to spinal ligaments that run in front of and behind the vertebral bodies. Tendons, which also connect muscles in the spine, can develop inflammation, or tendonitis.

Muscles in the back can strain or spasm and become a hard lump, much like a charley horse in a leg. Back muscle spasms can be caused by injury and pain, whether the source is muscle strain or a disc problem. A spasm, an involuntary convulsive contraction of muscle fibers, can be excruciating. The muscle spasm may be steady, or come in waves of contractions. In a sense, your muscle is sending you a signal that you have pushed it beyond its ability to perform.

It is natural for a person to stop moving an injured area when they feel pain, and wait for it to heal. Ironically, this is counterproductive. Restricting movement causes the muscle to weaken further, become less flexible, and receive less healing circulation. In fact, gentle stretching and exercise is the best and fastest way to resolve the injury by getting it moving and increasing circulation.

Vertebra Diagram

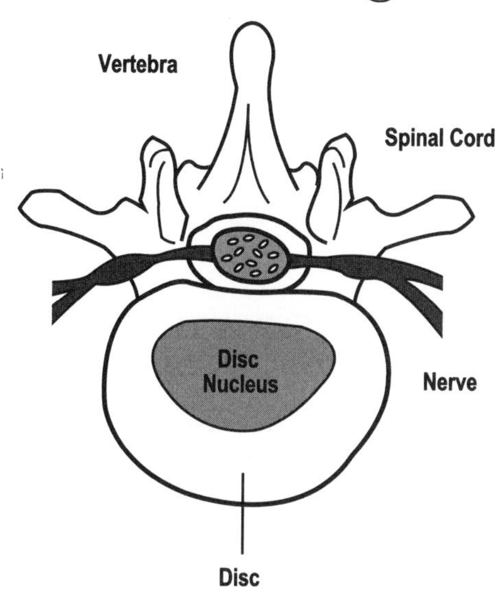

Above: *Cross section of the spine from above showing a "normal" disc.*

Below: *Cross section showing a herniated or ruptured disc. The disc herniation breaks through the disc wall and presses against the nerve, causing pain.*

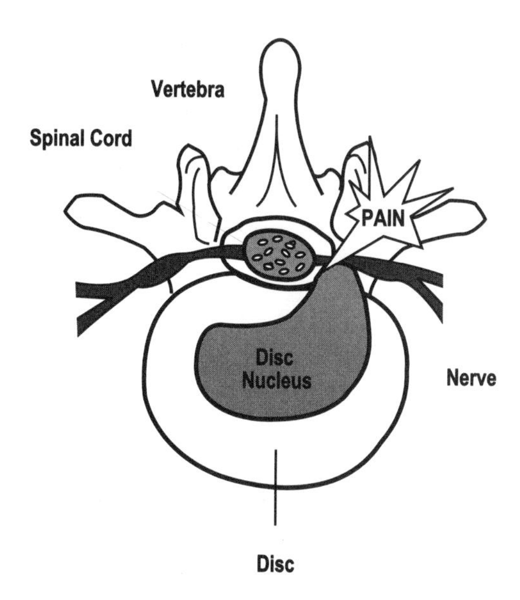

What is the difference between a sprain and a strain? While someone may argue that the two words are different, that a sprain is a more serious injury than a strain, in reality sprain and strain have evolved to mean essentially the same things to doctors and lawyers. Both words relate to an overworked muscle, or a ligament or tendon that is overstretched.

Some may argue that strain relates to stretching or tearing of muscles or tendons, while sprain relates to tearing of ligaments or tissues in a joint area. For example, if bones in a joint are forced beyond a comfortable range of motion, the joint may be sprained.

Another term that you may hear is "muscle spasm," where a muscle locks up in an excruciating, hard lump.

What is the difference between a simple strain and a herniated disc? Most people erroneously think that the more excruciating the pain, the more likely that you herniated a disc. That is not the case at all. In some cases a back spasm can cause excruciating pain, but if it is mostly in the lower back, it is probably not a herniated disc. A herniated disc in your back will typically radiate pain down into your leg, while a blown disc in your neck will radiate pain down your arm.

Disc herniation Once we reach our 20s the discs in the spine essentially stop receiving a blood supply. As we age, the discs can become brittle and more prone to degeneration. Exercise is like a lubricant for the discs, keeping them more pliant and resistant to herniation. Living a sedentary lifestyle and then lifting a heavy object one day can cause a disc to herniate. Often times, back pain without leg pain can be from a partial herniation of the disc, or an internal disc disruption.

Facet joint pain The facet joints act as hinges in our backs, enabling the spinal vertebrae to move and twist. Sometimes degeneration of the joint, perhaps from arthritis, may cause the facet joint to crack, much like a rusty hinge. Each facet joint has a capsule of lubricant, called synovial fluid, that keeps the joint moving freely. Sometimes the lining of the joint swells and becomes painfully irritated, just like a shoulder or elbow joint can become irritated and sore from too much tennis. Sometimes facet joint pain can be triggered by bending backwards.

Facet joint pain may be treated with anti-inflammatory drugs and gentle exercise. Even so, you should avoid bending in a way that may make it worse. If drugs and therapy don't work, sometimes injections may be required.

Whiplash Whiplash is a neck-specific injury often associated with a car accident. Whiplash occurs when the body stops suddenly while the weight of the head is going forward, stretching the muscles and tendons in the neck, and then the head snaps backward. While whiplash can be excruciating, and one would think the damage done from a car accident would require surgery, whiplash usually just causes muscle and ligament strain.

Although neck injuries of this sort can be quite painful, it is rare for whiplash to herniate a disc or fracture a vertebra. So, despite what it sounds like or what an attorney may say, whiplash is usually no more than a severe muscle strain in the neck. This does not mean it is easy to treat. Like any muscle strain, whiplash can require physical therapy for pain relief, and then a reconditioning program.

Back problems that may require surgery

Traumatic injury Perhaps the greatest trauma or damage to the back is caused by a car accident or a fall. Not only does this event usually catch the person by surprise, but it can cause more extensive damage to the back than lifting something heavy.

A serious injury to a specific level of vertebrae can effectively interrupt the electrical messages being sent from the brain to other parts of the body, resulting in paralysis.

The force of a fall can also crack vertebrae or herniate discs. In such traumatic accidents, surgery may be unavoidable. Any fracture of a vertebrae can require surgery to stabilize the spinal column because of the risk of more serious damage to the delicate spinal cord.

Disc-related problems The shock-absorbing discs that separate the bones in the spine are probably the most common reason for spine surgery. A disc is much like a jelly doughnut, in that it has an outside wall and a soft center. The "jelly" is the inner spongy portion of the disc, called the *nucleus pulposus*. Encircling the jelly-like nucleus are hard bands of fibrous tissue called the *annulus fibrosis*, or disc wall. Years of strain and poor form when lifting can take a toll. One day, a sudden stress from lifting a heavy package can cause a weakened disc to rupture, allowing the jelly center to squirt out of the disc space. This jelly contains chemicals which are extremely irritating to the nerves, which can also cause swelling.

Because the nerve roots act as telegraph lines to other parts of the body, a common complication of disc herniation is that it can cause pain that is felt in other parts of the body, like the leg. In fact, leg pain below the knee is a common symptom of a herniated disc.

This radiating pain is called radicular pain or radiculopathy. Unlike muscles, which can heal somewhat quickly, a torn or degenerated disc heals quite slowly. The good news is that, in many cases, the pain and inflammation originating from damaged discs can be treated non-surgically by reducing the inflammation and by strengthening the musculature surrounding the damaged disc to give it more support.

While herniated discs are often referred to as "slipped discs," this really isn't accurate. Discs are actually attached by connective tissue to the vertebrae above and below and so don't ever slip out of position. A disc herniation may be "contained" or "uncontained." With a bulge that is contained, for example, the jelly center remains within the disc wall. Uncontained means that some of the jelly nucleus has broken through the disc wall, but is still attached to the rest of the nucleus pulposus. A herniation may be "sequestered," when a part actually breaks free or separates from the rest of the nucleus and travels away from the disc.

Discs can herniate in any direction: forward, centrally, or — most commonly — backward and sideways in the direction of the spinal nerves.

Herniated discs account for a small percentage of back pain. Normal disc degeneration which naturally occurs with old age can also cause pain.

In summary, it is important that you not overreact when a physician or radiologist finds a herniated disc on an x-ray, CT scan, or MRI. Sometimes even healthy people without back or neck pain have disc problems. Even if your disc problem is causing your pain, there is a lot you can do to relieve your symptoms non-surgically.

Scoliosis Some people are born with, or develop over time, abnormal curves in their spine. This may cause the person to be bent over, or have a slight hump in their back. This curvature, referred to as scoliosis, involves the spine not just bending, but rather twisting like a bent corkscrew.

No one knows what causes scoliosis. It happens more with females than males, and there is nothing anyone can do to prevent it from appearing. If it does appear, doctors may try to use a brace to prevent the curve from worsening.

In some cases of scoliosis, if the curve is bad enough, it may put pressure on the internal organs. This may shorten life expectancy and surgery may be required. Scoliosis surgery is extremely complex, and a person should invest a great deal of time in selecting an orthopedic surgeon who sub-specializes in using the most current surgical fixation rods. If a surgeon tries to correct the curve too much, or uses an improper method, the person could be paralyzed from the surgery.

Lordosis and kyphosis Other spinal deformities involve other types of abnormal curves in the spine. When the spine curves too much inward in the lower back, it is called lordosis. When the spine in the shoulder blade area has too much forward curve, or too much of a hump, it is called kyphosis.

Spinal stenosis Stenosis is caused by the spinal canal not being large enough for the spinal nerves, much like a ring that can cut off the circulation on a swollen finger. The problem may come from a vertebral area that crimps the spinal nerves, causing swelling and discomfort. It is a condition that may appear as a person gets older.

The symptoms include a deep aching in the lower back, buttocks and thigh, and radiating shock-like pains in the legs, which may feel heavy and useless. The symptoms can be brought on by walking and exercise. If you have stenosis, you may notice that pain is sometimes relieved by sitting, or by a position where the spine is flexed forward and bending over. Consequently, people with stenosis may walk with a stooped over posture, and are able to sit without symptoms. Conversely, people with stenosis may find that their pain gets worse when they bend backward.

In many cases, changing posture and using spinal injections can control the symptoms for a long period of time. Stenosis is an ailment that may appear as a person gets older. In some cases, surgery is needed to widen the passageway for the spinal cord.

Arthritis Just as stenosis is a problem associated with growing older, so is arthritis, a disease that causes degeneration of joints. Arthritis can manifest itself as a narrowing of the spinal canal (stenosis) or as facet joint problems in the back. As with other forms of arthritis that affect hands, shoulders and knees, it can be difficult to treat back pain from arthritis.

Osteoporosis Another problem associated with old age is osteoporosis. Osteoporosis is a gradual weakening of bone density and strength. It typically comes on without any symptoms, and mostly affects older women. Often a woman will be unaware she has the problem until a bone fracture occurs. In the back, osteoporosis can put a person at risk of a vertebral fracture. If your physician suspects that you have osteoporosis, you may need a type of bone scan to reveal how porous your bones may be. Sometimes dietary supplements or medication may be recommended to address the problem.

Spondylolysis and spondylolisthesis These problems relate to instability in specific bones in the lower back. As you recall, the rear part of spinal vertebrae have facet joints that act as hinges, allowing our spines to twist and bend. Sometimes, either from heredity or from wear and tear, a specific part of the posterior element called the pars interarticularis cracks. This can let the vertebrae slip forward out of its correct position.

Spondylolysis occurs when the pars hinge is cracked but the vertebra is still in its correct position. Spondylolisthesis occurs when the cracked pars has allowed the vertebra to slide forward out of its correct position.

Gymnasts, for example, who perform routines that bend and arch the back are often victims of spondylolysis or spondylolisthesis.

While ligaments and muscles can help hold the vertebra in place, surgery may become necessary over time, to install surgical instrumentation or bone grafts that lock the vertebra in place so it doesn't slide out of position and damage the spinal nerves. Interestingly, in many cases, spondylolisthesis may have no symptoms, so most people may not know they have it. If back pain doesn't go away on its own over a few weeks, a spine doctor will check for such instability through x-rays or other diagnostic test.

Notes

1. "Abnormal Magnetic Resonance Scans of the Lumber Spine in Asymptomatic Subjects." *Journal of Bone & Joint Surgery* 72-A no. 3 (March 1990).
2. "Low Back Pain Hospitalization — Recent United States Trends and Regional Variations." *Spine* 19 no. 11 (1994): 1207–12 .

PART 2

Back Care and Treatment

CHAPTER 3

Mainstream Ways to Treat Your Back on Your Own

Twenty years ago, the most common treatment for back pain was bed rest. A person complaining of extreme back pain would end up hospitalized, essentially being placed on forced bed rest. A lot of orthopedic problems, sore arms, broken wrists, and strained ankles were treated with traction, casts, and slings that immobilized the injury for several months.

About that time, sports medicine experts who treated injured athletes started to challenge the conventional medical wisdom. Athletes couldn't wait several months or years for something to heal, and then begin a long recovery and rehabilitation process to re-strengthen all the muscles that had become de-conditioned and weak from inactivity. Consequently, physicians started rehabilitation sooner and sooner. Soon the philosophy changed from immobilization to "get the patient moving as soon as possible."

An important general rule of thumb about back and neck pain, as well as using a home remedy: if your back or neck pain symptoms start to get worse over a few days, visit your back physician. Chapter 7 provides more detail on when you need to see a doctor.

First aid remedies for back pain

Step 1: Ice then heat Remember this rule for any strain or sprain: ice then heat. The reason is that right after an injury, there will be inflammation. You want to reduce that inflammation by applying ice to the injured area. Ice makes the blood vessels in that area constrict, which reduces blood flow and reduces initial swelling.

But after 48 hours or so, you want to begin using heat to actually increase the flow of blood to the affected area, which will increase healing.

Also remember to never apply ice for more than five minutes at a time because it can freeze the skin and cause soft tissue damage. The same for heat, which can also do damage if applied for too long.

A good tip for back and neck pain is to take several paper cups, fill them with water, and place them in the freezer. Once they are frozen, peel back the paper edge, leaving a paper handle. Then let your partner apply the ice to the sore area for five minutes at a time.

Step 2: Anti-inflammatories You can find everything you need to resolve simple back and neck pain at the local drug store. The best drugs for back and neck pain are anti-inflammatory drugs called "non-steroidal anti-inflammatory drugs" or, as you will often see abbreviated by physicians, NSAIDs.

The most common NSAIDs are ibuprofen products like Advil or Nuprin. If you are allergic to these medications, you can try naproxyn sodium which is found in products like Aleve, or acetaminophen found in Tylenol, or try aspirin.

Remember, if you have an attack of back pain, start the medication and keep taking it for a few days as directed on the bottle. This will provide a constant level of the drug in your body. It is less effective to take a couple of pills, let them wear off, and the next day start again.

Generally speaking, the best anti-inflammatory for back pain is ibuprofen, and the next best is aspirin. Acetaminophen as an analgesic is geared to reduce pain and fever rather than inflammation, but it can be used by those people who cannot take aspirin or ibuprofen because of stomach irritation.

It is important to have a basic understanding of how various over-the-counter medications work. The body has a group of internal chemicals called prostaglandins. When you hurt yourself, prostaglandins are released and excite nerve endings, which you feel as pain. NSAIDs provide pain relief primarily by inhibiting prostaglandins throughout your body. NSAIDs may irritate your stomach lining, however, and so you may not be able to take them. If you have an irritable stomach or an ulcer, consult your doctor. He or she may recommend an alternative medication which contains acetaminophen. This provides pain relief by working on the central nervous system, and does not affect your stomach.

If you are already taking any sort of pill for another problem, or if you have any other existing medical problem in addition to your back or neck pain, you should always *consult your physician before self-medicating. There can be dangerous side effects from taking two medications together. Also, you should follow the directions on the bottle carefully. Taking too much of a medicine, or taking it for too many days, can cause serious problems.*

Remember: Drugs do not act on the source of the pain, such as a strained muscle. Drugs typically reduce the pain and allow you to begin flexibility exercises that help relax the muscle and make it more mobile.

Step 3: Relax, but limit your bed rest to 2 days An attack of back pain is a signal from your body to your brain that you did something wrong. Listen to the signal and stop what you're doing. If you are playing a round of golf, stop swinging. Walk the rest of the round, or walk into the clubhouse and call it a day. If you are at work, let your supervisor know that you hurt your back.

If your back strain is severe enough, you may end up in bed. But limit your bed rest to two days. Any more inactivity causes muscles to atrophy. For example, if you ever injure a limb and have it immobilized in a cast for several weeks, that limb will be very stiff after the cast is removed. The muscles weaken, become less flexible, and are resistant to movement. The same thing happens after a back pain attack. People naturally restrict their movement to prevent additional pain, but restricting movement can make recovery that much more difficult. For that matter, any back pain that is so severe that you have to stay in bed at all probably needs to be looked at by a physician.

Step 4: Walk If you can tolerate it, just getting up and walking around the neighborhood is good for your back. A walk gets you moving, gets the blood flowing, and begins to stretch out stiff muscles. It can also relieve some of the tension which may be making your back pain worse. For people who are overweight, however, even walking may be difficult because of the loads placed on the spine. If walking sounds or feels difficult, consider walking in a pool. The water creates an artificial semi-weightlessness, so even heavy people find it easier and less painful. The slower you walk the easier it is, and if you want more resistance, you can try walking faster. The water can also feel therapeutic.

Exercise

For a back pain sufferer, advice to get moving again may seem aggressive. Research has shown clearly, however, that activity is the best medicine for acute back pain. In 1997, Britain's highly respected Royal College of General Practitioners released national clinical guidelines for managing acute back pain. The guidelines stress that in the absence of red flags like trauma, loss of control of the bowel or bladder, or weakness in a leg, back pain will resolve faster with a gradual increase in activity, rather than bed rest.

As to how active to be and how fast to return to activity, the Royal College advises patients to "let pain be your guide."

How does exercise work? Because many discs herniate or bulge toward the back side of the spine, extension exercises, where the back is arched backward slightly, are thought to relieve pressure on the front side of the disc, which may in turn create a vacuum that draws the herniation back in slightly. Remember that these exercises are not repairing the damaged disc, though they may help make disc symptoms go away.

Exercises that relieve pain Few people have impacted the profession of back care more than Robin McKenzie, a physical therapist from New Zealand. His special set of bending and stretching exercises has had dramatic results, and can take someone with excruciating back strain and move them in the span of minutes to a pain-free state. Before McKenzie, drugs, physical therapy modalities, chiropractic, and surgery were the standard treatments for back pain. McKenzie, in many ways, pioneered the use of special exercises to relieve pain and make symptoms disappear.

How exercise can help a herniated disc

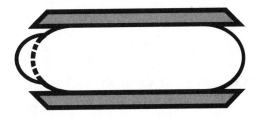

The saucers illustrated above sandwich a water balloon in the same way that two vertebrae sandwich the soft intervertebral disc. The bulge on the left side of the balloon represents a disc herniation.

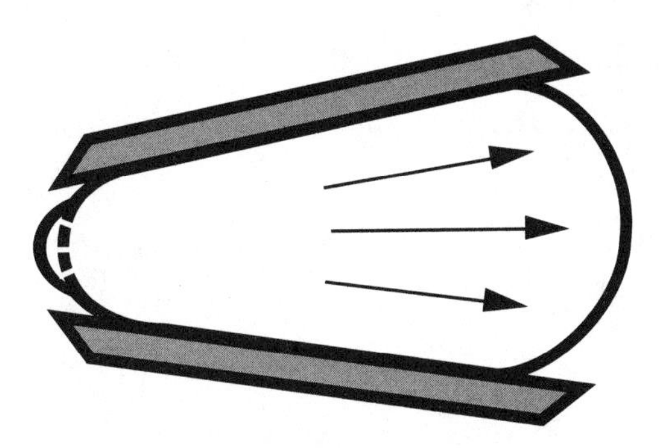

Through special extension exercises (starting on page 39) that arch the back and tilt both vertebrae, the disc is compressed on the side with the herniation. The theory is that compressing the side with the herniation lessens the pressure on the front side of the disc, which creates a vacuum. This vacuum may then draw the herniation back inward, lessening the painful pressure on the nearby nerve root. The result: the disc herniation has not been fixed, but the pain generated by the herniated disc is lessened.

Today, there are widely accepted sets of exercises that many spine centers recommend for relief of simple back pain. And yes, exercises can really relieve an attack of back pain. While it is hard for a back pain sufferer to believe that further movement of the injured area will actually help rather than hurt, the specific exercises shown in this chapter *can* relieve pain symptoms.

What you can do on your own vs. with a therapist Many therapy centers look a lot like fitness centers. In fact, more physical therapists are starting to include free weights in their rehab centers because working with free weights more closely resembles activities of daily living than do workout machines. So, if you belong to a gym, once you are over your initial pain episode there is a lot you can do to treat yourself without going to a therapist.

Large companies are following this trend. Apple Computer, Electronic Data Systems, General Motors, Texas Instruments, Northern Telecom (Nortel) all bring physical therapists into their fitness facilities to enable their corporate fitness areas to do double duty. At General Motors' Powertrain Division, about 50 percent of the employees with worker's compensation injuries are rehabilitated through the company's fitness center. Using a fitness club also returns the worker to an active lifestyle more successfully. General Motors reports that, since 1994, the number of workers out on disability has dropped from about 70 to 25. This represents a savings to GM in 1995 of $250,000 in worker time and $50,000 in medical costs.

Pool exercises Water is your best friend when recovering from back or neck strain. That is because, after an attack of back or neck pain, even walking around can be painful. Water is therapeutic, and it creates a kind of artificial weightlessness. Walking in a pool is sort of like walking on the moon. It is less jarring, and your body weight is somewhat decreased by the water's buoyancy. However, the faster you try to walk in a pool, the more resistance you create, which makes it a perfect progressive resistance exercise device. You can even wear hydrotherapy fins on your hands to increase the resistance of your arms as they move through the water.

For anyone who has endured the searing drop-to-your-knees back pain attack, by far the biggest fear is of doing anything that may cause a recurrence. By starting in water you can build flexibility and strength in a non-threatening way, and then gradually build up to working out with exercise machines.

Neck pain sufferers should avoid swimming initially because of the strain on the neck when doing the crawl.

Building your own home treatment program Some of the exercises shown in this section (starting on page 39) can be effective home remedies for an attack of back or neck pain in that they can actually relieve pain symptoms. Those exercises are noted accordingly. There are other exercises that strengthen the back and make it more flexible. Still other exercises are especially helpful to those active in sports, especially rotational sports like tennis or golf that place heavy demands on the back.

You will notice that the exercises are grouped into those that involve lying on the floor, and those that can be done standing up. The floor exercises are best for doing at home or at the gym before you move into more aggressive workouts. The standing exercises can be done at work, on the golf course, in an aisle on the plane, in a highway rest area, or any time during the day when you want to give your back a time out.

Here are some basic guidelines for doing the exercises. Don't hold your breath when exercising; breathe normally. Stretch slowly, not abruptly, and never to the point of causing sharp pain. Remember, it took years for your muscles to shorten and become less flexible. It will take months of stretching to lengthen them out again. Make a point of noticing, for example, how far you can stretch the first time you start these exercises. Then note again after a month or so. You will probably see your body begin to stretch farther as the muscles and tendons become more flexible.

When you count, count "one Mississippi, two Mississippi," etc. Stretching exercises are done slowly, to give the muscle an opportunity to gently stretch out. You may notice that some days are easier than others. That is normal. On the days that you feel unusually stiff or sore, take it easy.

Never bounce or jerk abruptly during your stretches. The correct motion is slow and steady, not bouncy or jerky.

You can use these exercises as many times during the day as you need them. If you have to sit at a desk a lot during the day, take a five-minute break every hour, stand, move around, and do some stretches to help your back out. You should try to dedicate a minimum of 30 minutes a day to work through a complete home exercise program. Some people like going through their program to start the day, others who are pressed for time in the morning prefer to go through their routine in the evening on the floor in front of the TV. Either way is good for your back.

Exercises to Relieve Back and Neck Pain

Exercises demonstrated by Shannon Hanlon
Exercise photos by Paul Buck

The authors extend their appreciation to

Steve Winkler, PT, Director of Rehabilitation at the Center for Spine, Savannah, Georgia, who provided his expertise on the exercises in this chapter.

Shannon Hanlon, personal trainer, winner of the West Coast Fitness Championship and Mid-USA Fitness Championship, and co-owner with husband Mark Hanlon of the Southlake Training Center, Southlake, Texas.

Exercise photos courtesy of Prizm Development, Inc.

Exercise 1:   Pain relieving extension

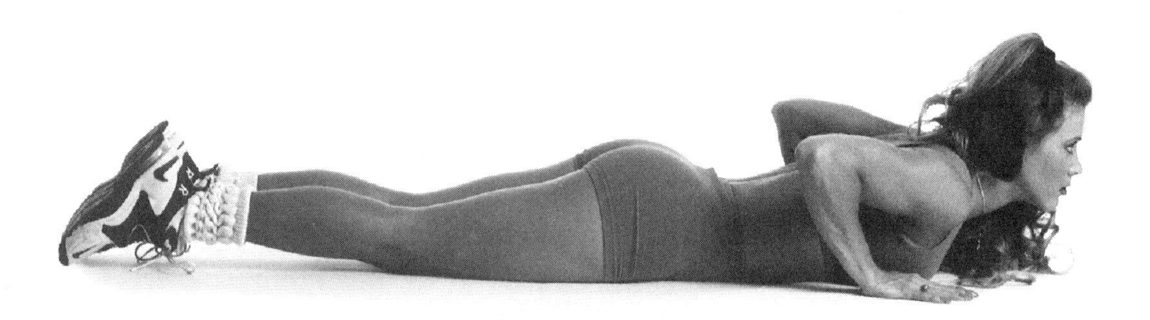

Level One

This exercise can be used as a first-aid remedy for simple back pain. Start by lying on your stomach, head down, then try to press up slightly, straightening your arms a little and raising your head to look straight in front. Keep your hips in contact with the floor and avoid tightening your lower back. The intent is *not* to do a push up with a straight back. Hold the arched position for ten seconds, then go back down to a lying position. Repeat five or ten times.

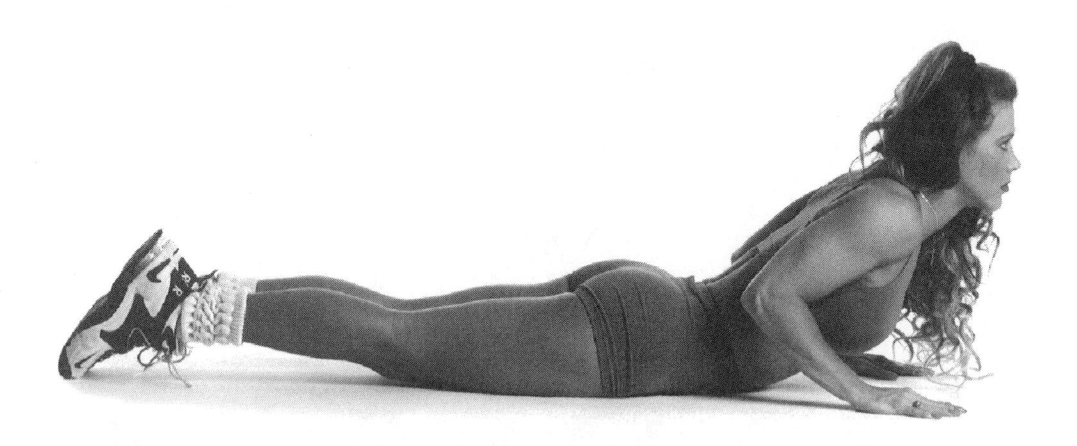

Level Two

Levels Two and Three involve raising the head and little more. There is a fourth level shown later that has the arms extended and locked completely, with the hips still pressed against the floor. This fourth position may be too difficult early on for someone with acute back pain. Stop if the pain becomes worse.

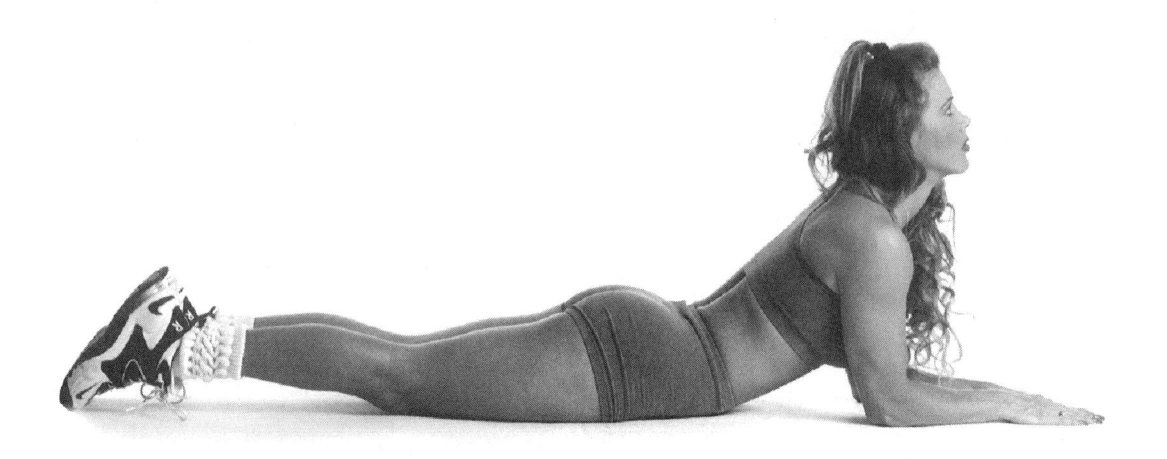

Level Three

Exercise 2: Pain relieving flexion *(1)*

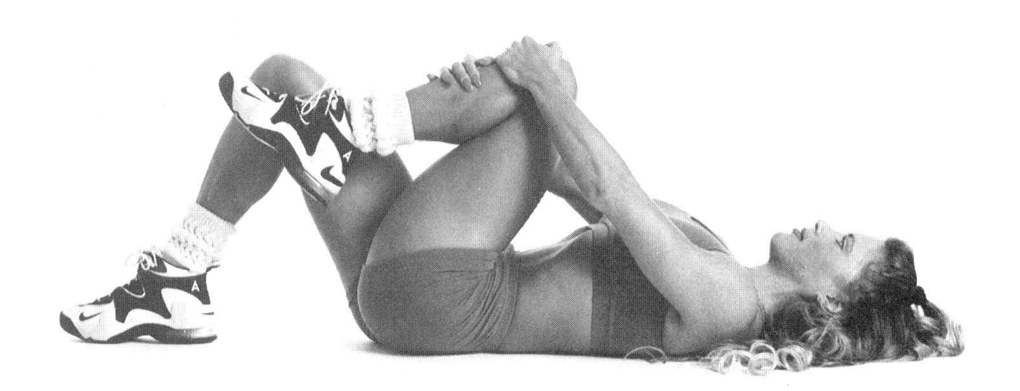

Lie on your back with both knees bent, feet flat on the floor. Lift one knee and bring it up toward your chest. Hold for ten seconds, then lower it to the starting position. Repeat with the other leg. As you progress with this exercise, start with both legs extended rather than with your knees bent.

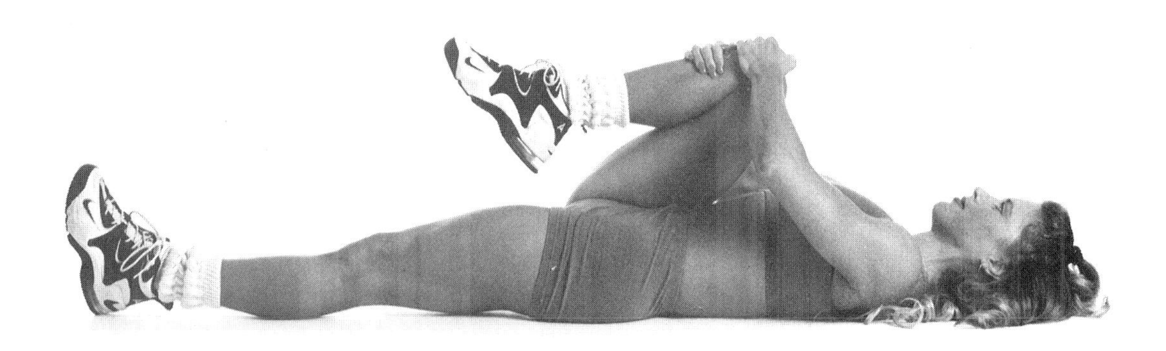

Exercise 3: Pain relieving flexion *(2)*

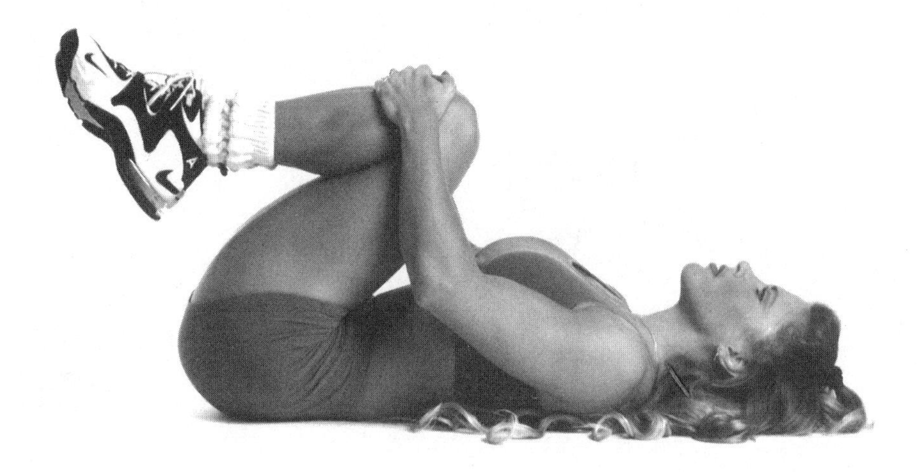

From the knees bent position with feet on the floor, bring both knees up toward your chest and hold for ten seconds. Repeat ten times. Increase the flexion as you are able, being sure to be guided by your pain at all times.

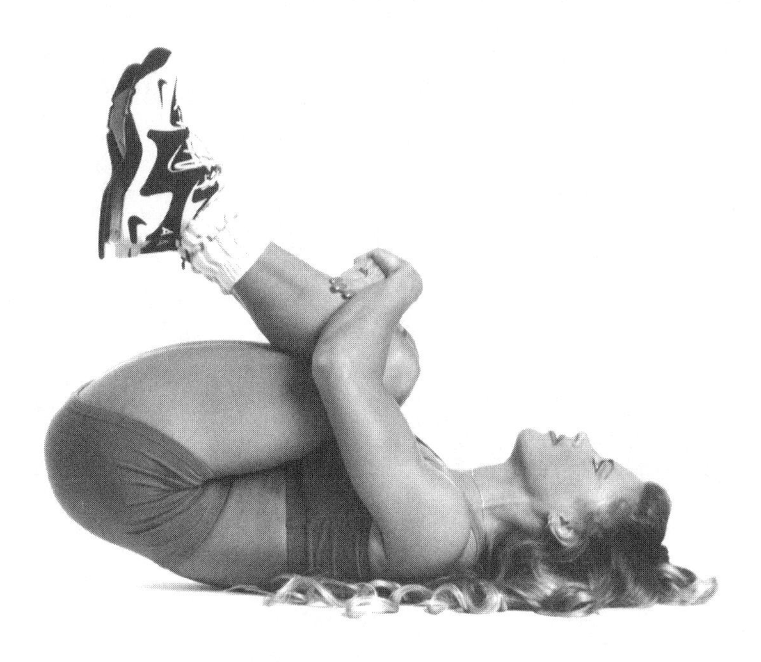

Exercise 4: Pain relieving lumbar rotation — single knee

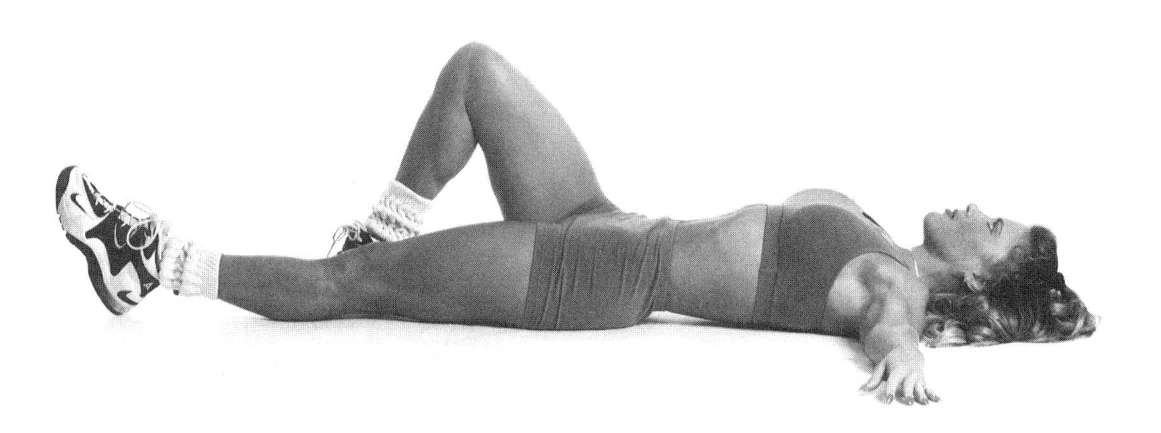

Lie flat on the floor on your back with your arms extended to the sides. Raise *one* knee and slowly cross it over your body, trying to let it touch the floor on the opposite side. Try to keep your shoulders flat against the ground. Hold for ten seconds, then go back to the starting position and repeat with your other knee. Do this ten times for each side.

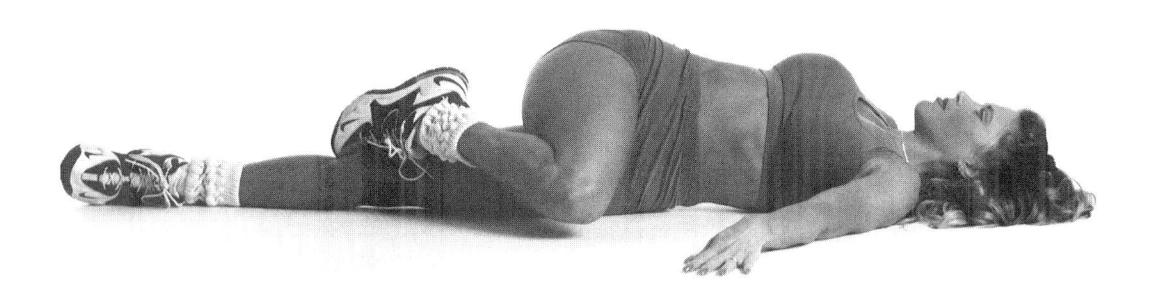

Exercise 5: Pain relieving lumbar rotation — double knee

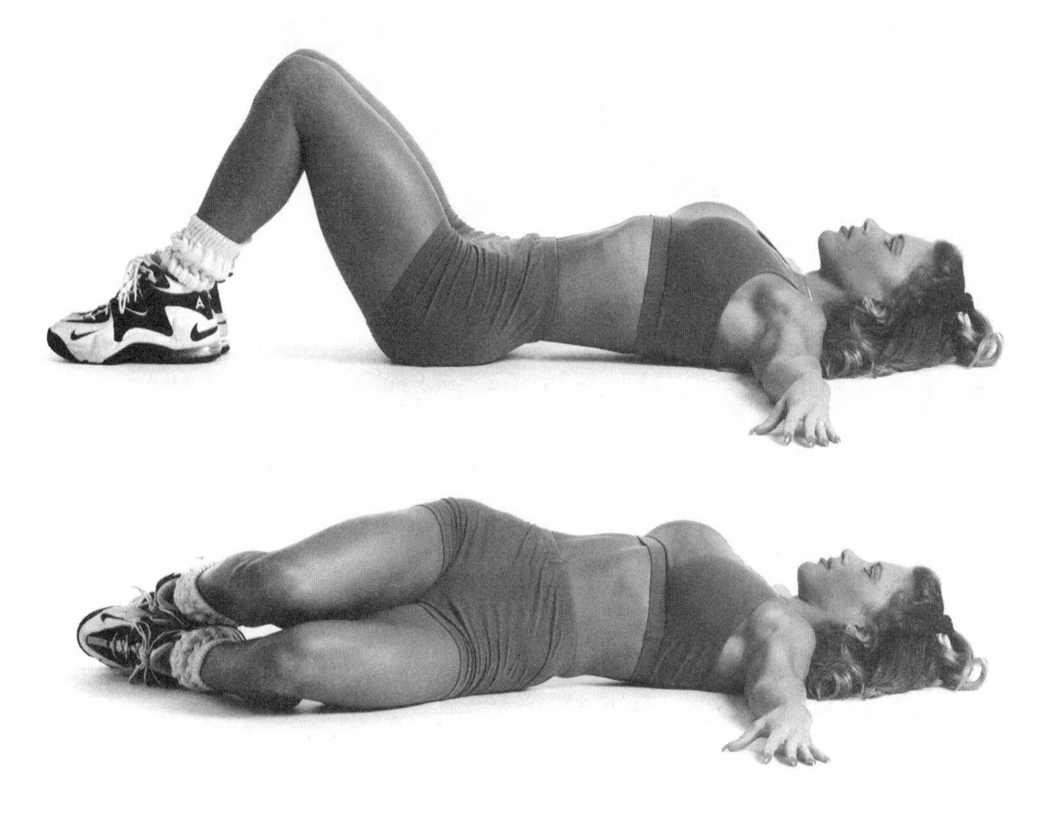

Raise both knees, keeping your feet flat on the floor, and slowly lower them to one side, trying to let them touch the floor. Try to keep your shoulders flat against the ground. Hold for ten seconds. Do this ten times for each side.

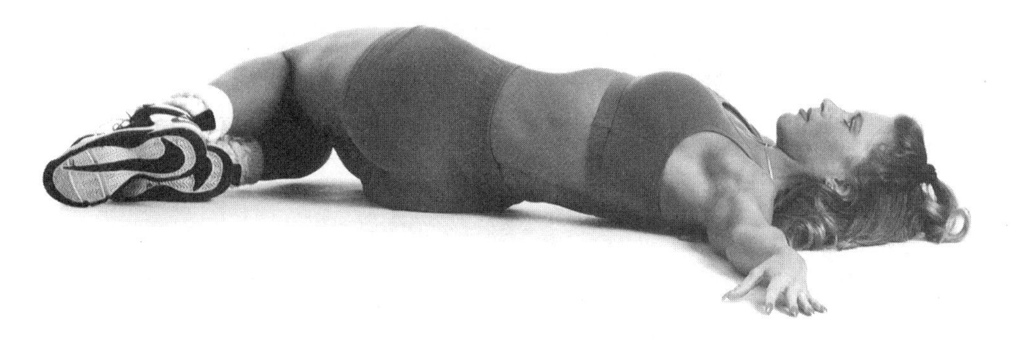

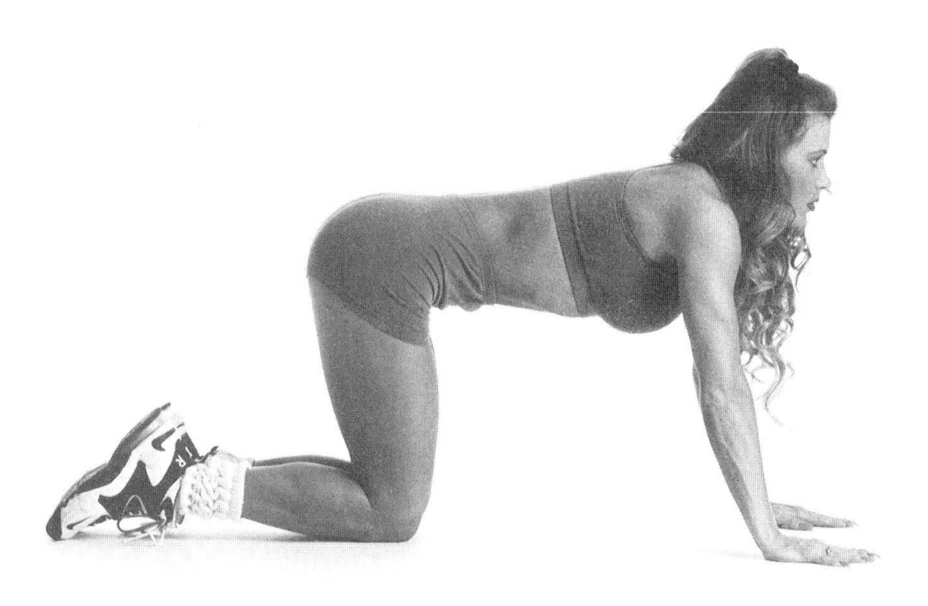

Exercise 6: Pain relieving lumbar flexion

From an all-fours position, knees on the ground, arch your lower back slightly and hold for ten seconds. Alternate between arching upward and downward. Repeat this up to twenty times.

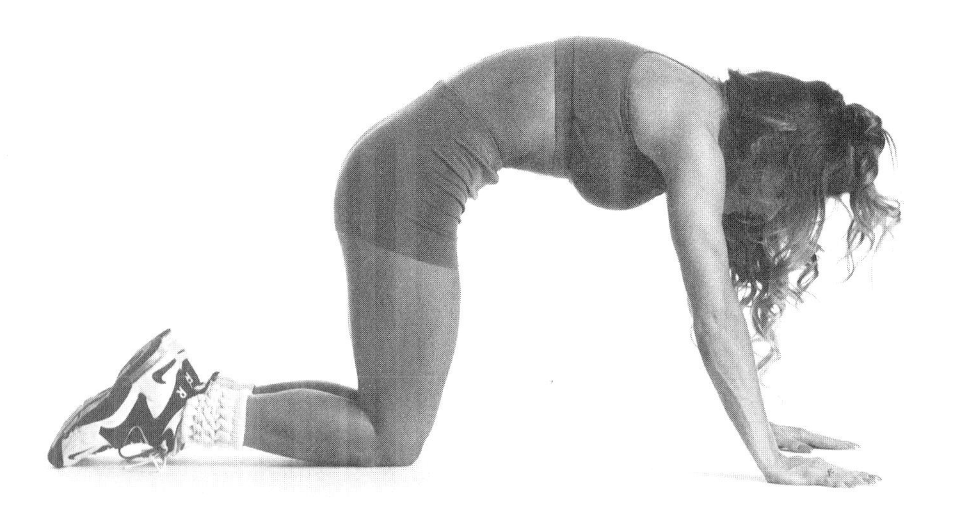

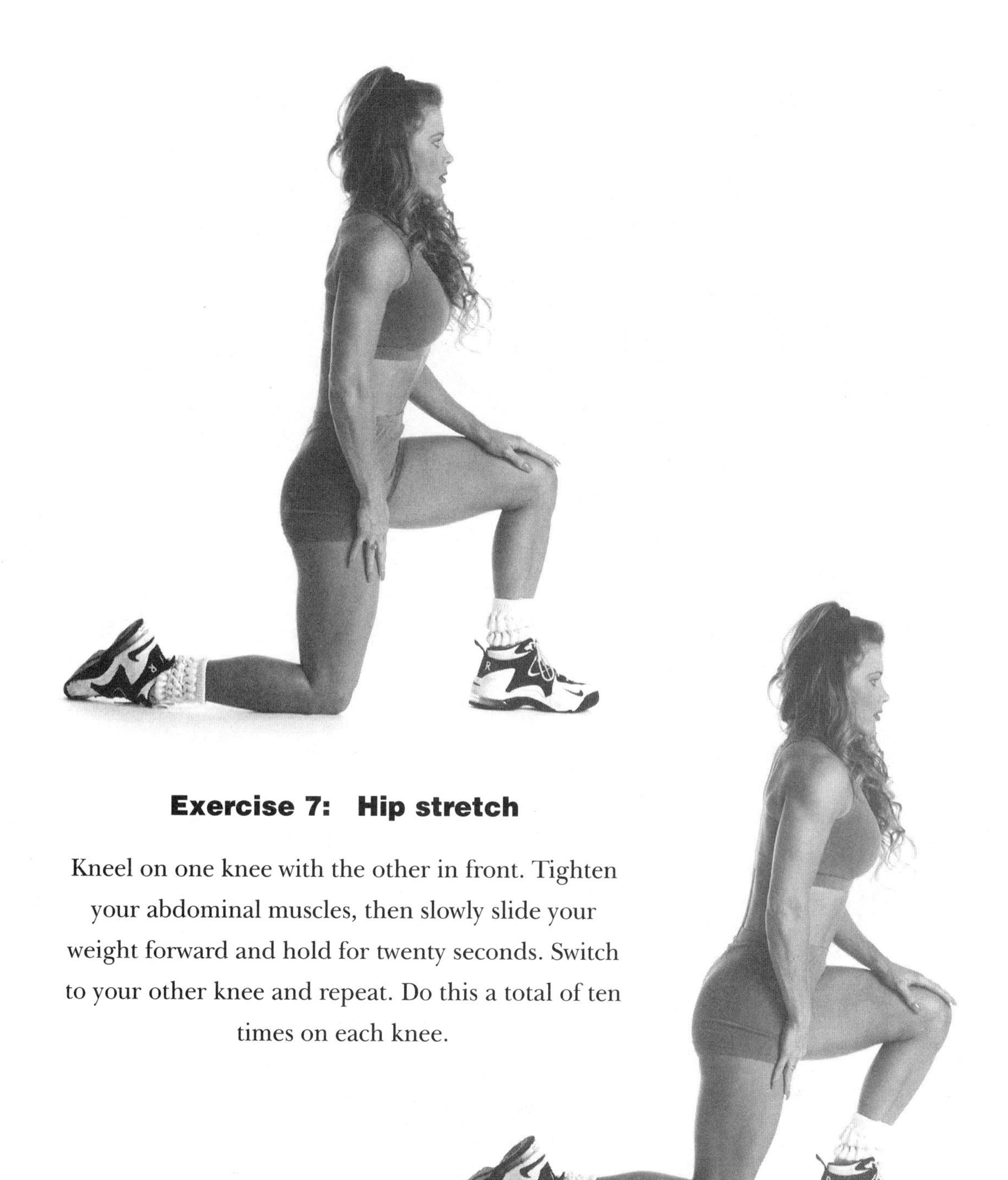

Exercise 7: Hip stretch

Kneel on one knee with the other in front. Tighten your abdominal muscles, then slowly slide your weight forward and hold for twenty seconds. Switch to your other knee and repeat. Do this a total of ten times on each knee.

Exercise 8: Abdominal strengthening diagonal curl

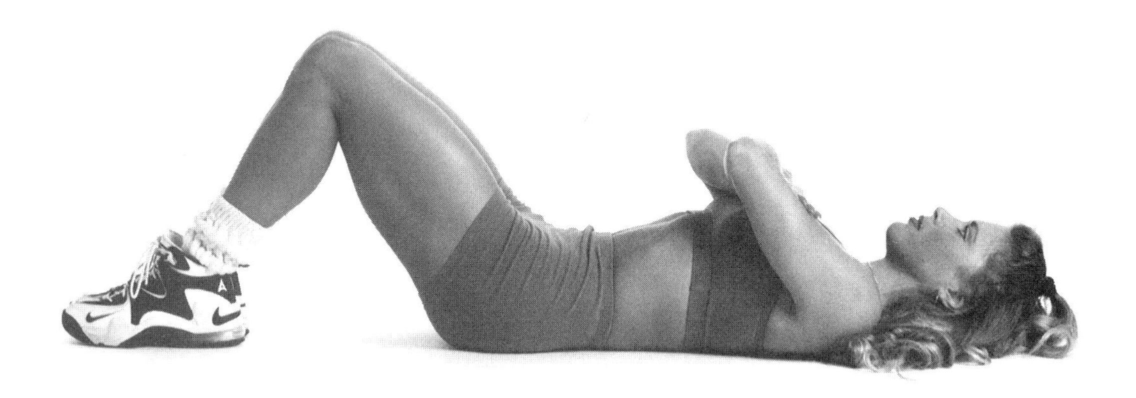

This exercise strengthens your abdominal muscles, which support and protect your back muscles from future strain. Lie on your back with knees bent, feet flat on the floor, and hands across the chest. (We don't advise putting your hands behind your head because it is possible to jerk your arms and hurt your neck in the process.) Do a partial sit up while pointing your right elbow at your left hip, then repeat to the other side. Repeat this twenty times.

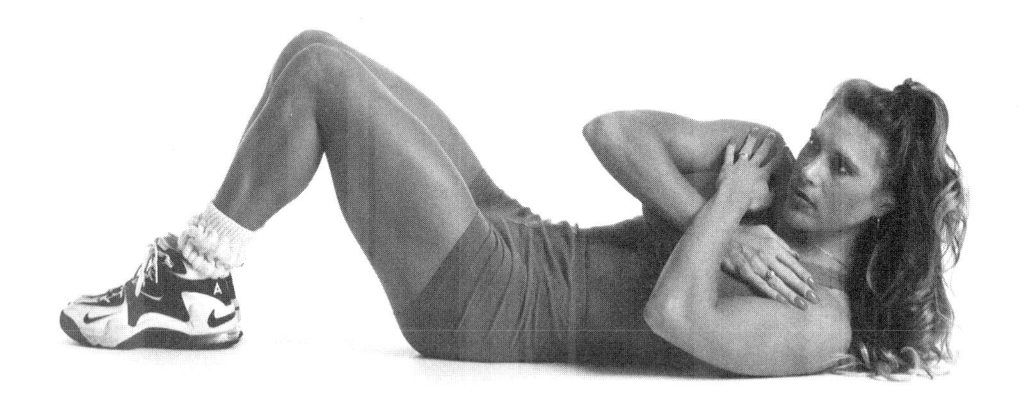

Exercise 9: Bridging

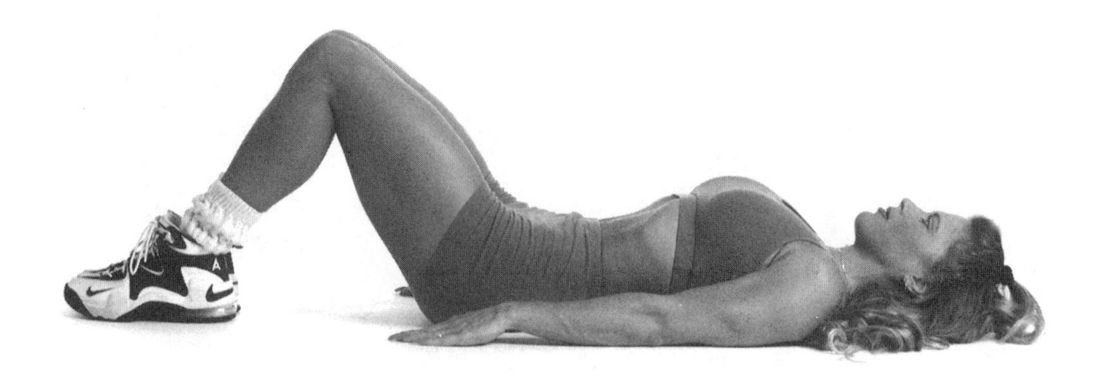

Lie flat on the floor on your back, arms by your sides, palms downward. Raise both your knees to a bent position, keeping your feet flat on the floor. Raise your hips up as far as you can without discomfort, then lower slowly to the starting position. Repeat this movement ten times.

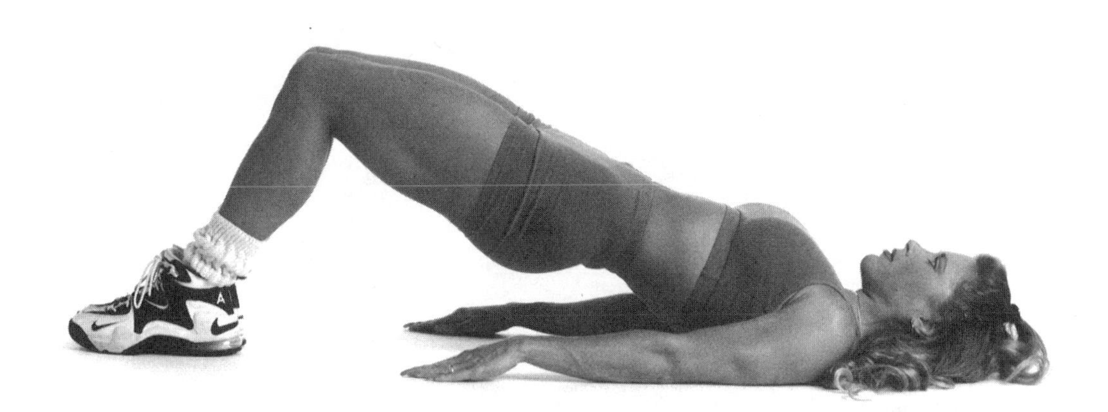

Exercise 10: Advanced press up

This is an advanced position of Exercise 1. Press up as before but extend to where the arms are fully straightened and locked. Hold for ten seconds, go back to the lying, resting position. Relax, and breathe deeply. Repeat ten times, with thirty seconds between each repetition.

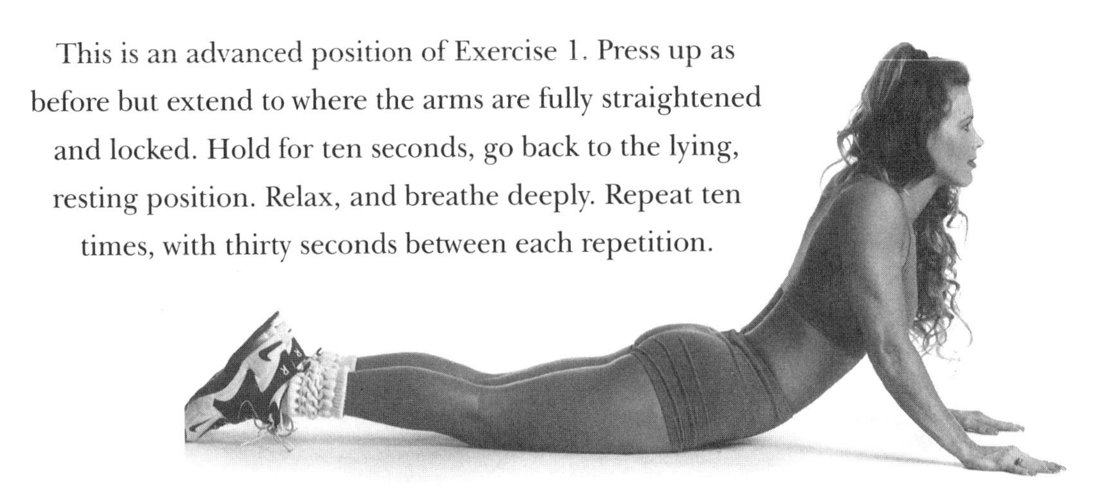

Exercise 11: Advanced stretch

This can be done in many variations with both hands on the ground and raising and extending one leg at a time. The advanced position, shown here, has the left leg raised and extended along with the right arm. Repeat by extending the right leg and left arm.

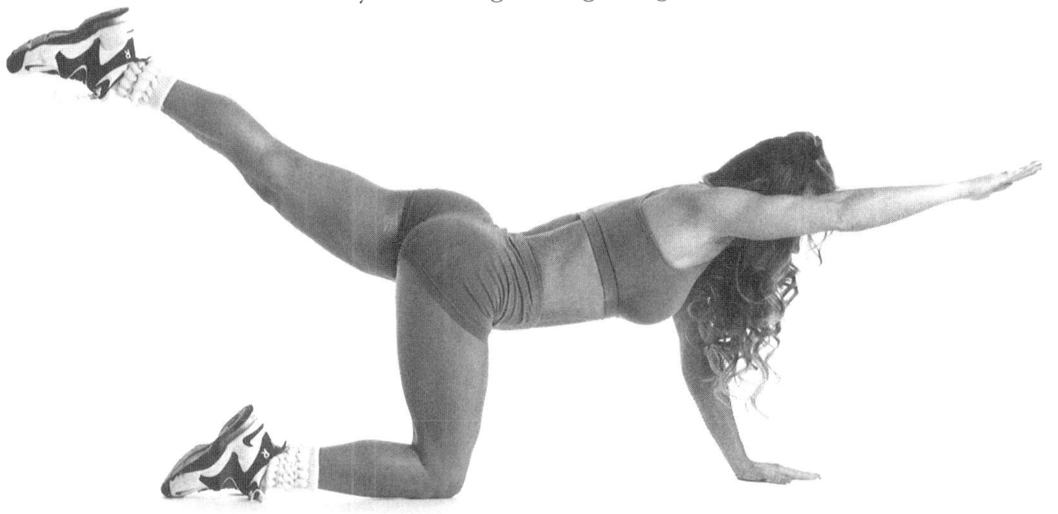

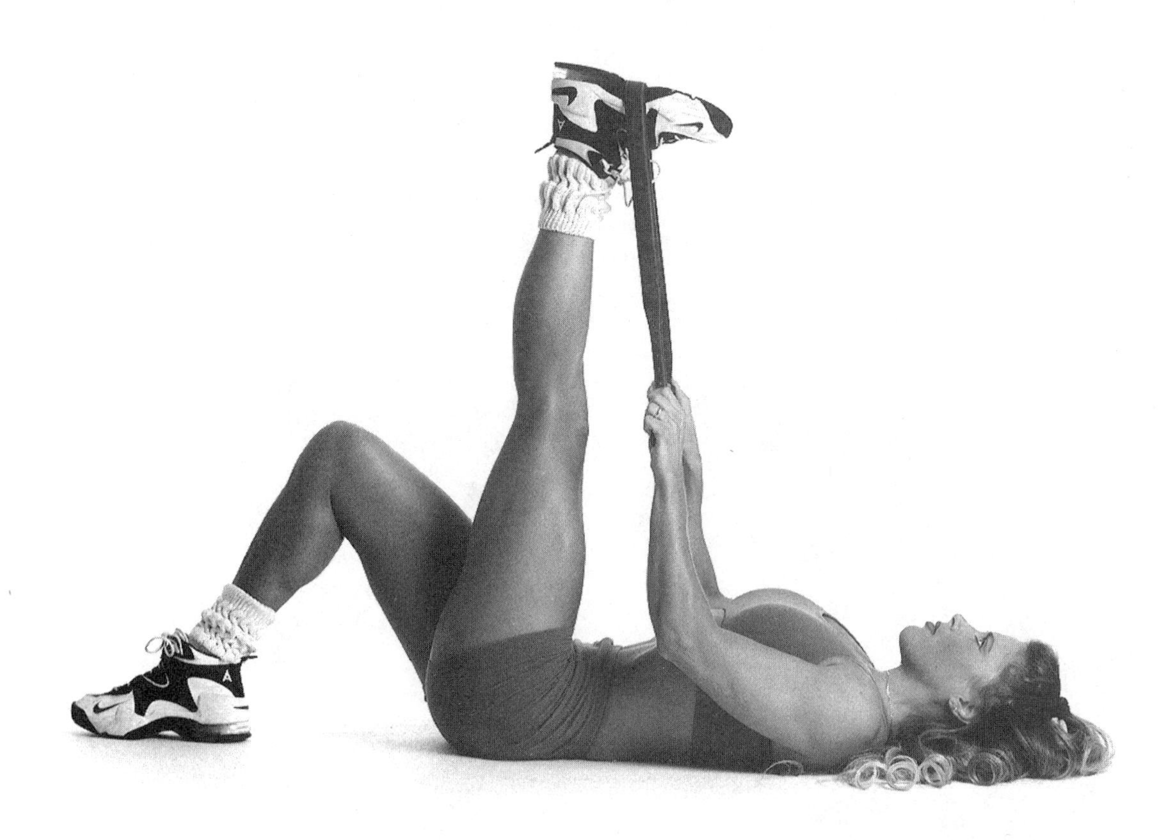

Exercise 12: Hamstring stretch

This exercise may not look hard, but try it — you may be surprised. Because most Americans spend so much time sitting behind a desk, our hamstrings (the muscles in the backs of our legs) tend to shorten and tighten over time. This exercise helps to increase flexibility. Lie flat on your back with one knee raised and that foot flat on the floor. With the other leg lying flat, and knee locked straight, take a belt and loop it around the instep of your foot. Slowly raise your leg as close as possible to a vertical position. Hold for thirty seconds and start over with your other leg.

Neck Exercises

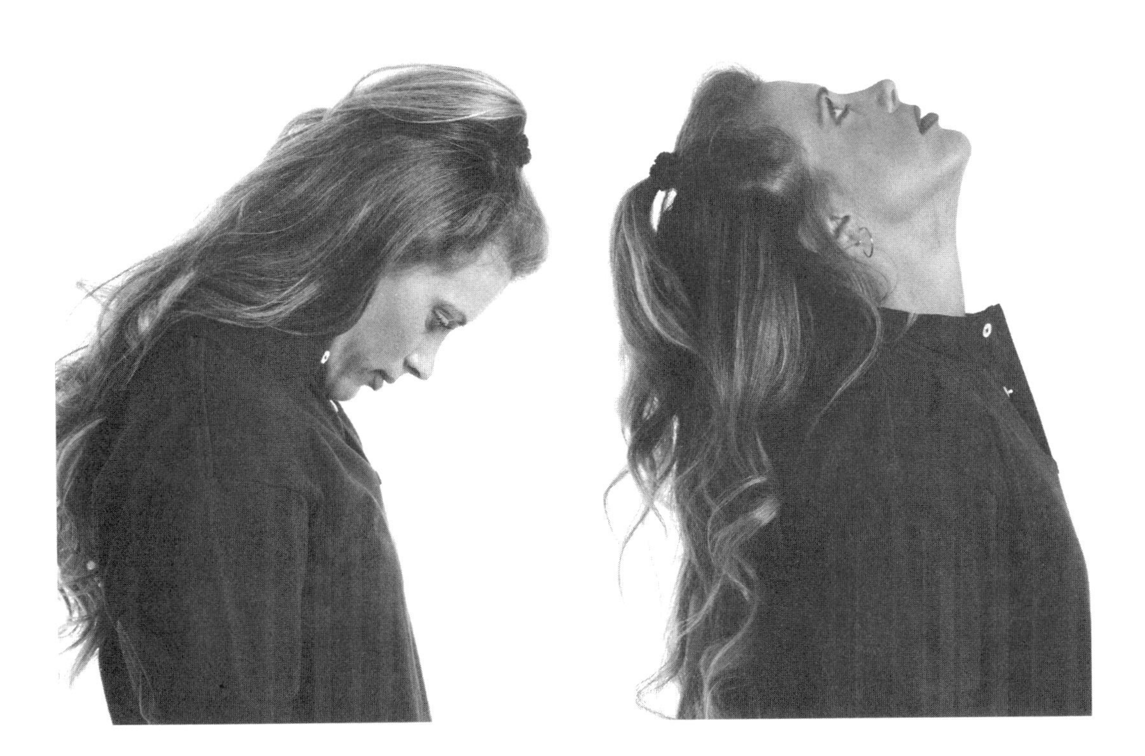

Exercise series 13: Neck stretches

From a starting neutral position, first stretch your neck downward (flexion) and then backward (extension). Hold each stretch position for ten seconds. Repeat ten times.

Neck stretches *(continued)*

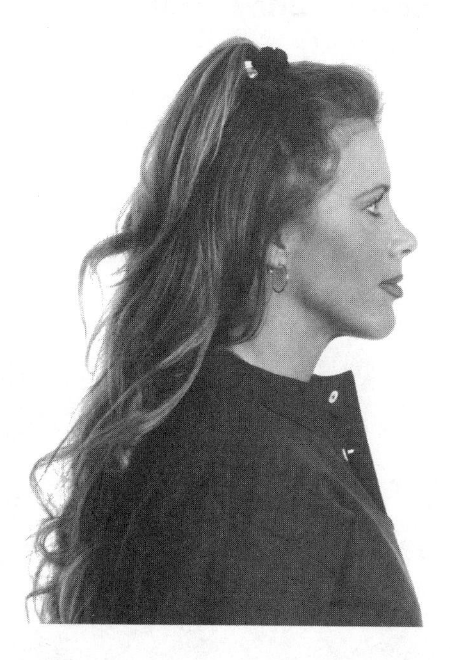

This is called a neck glide. From a starting neutral position slowly slide your chin forward and hold for ten seconds, then release. Repeat ten times.

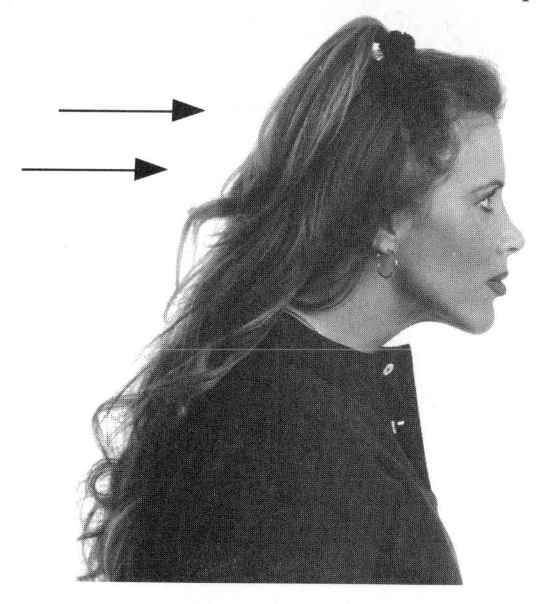

Neck stretches *(continued)*

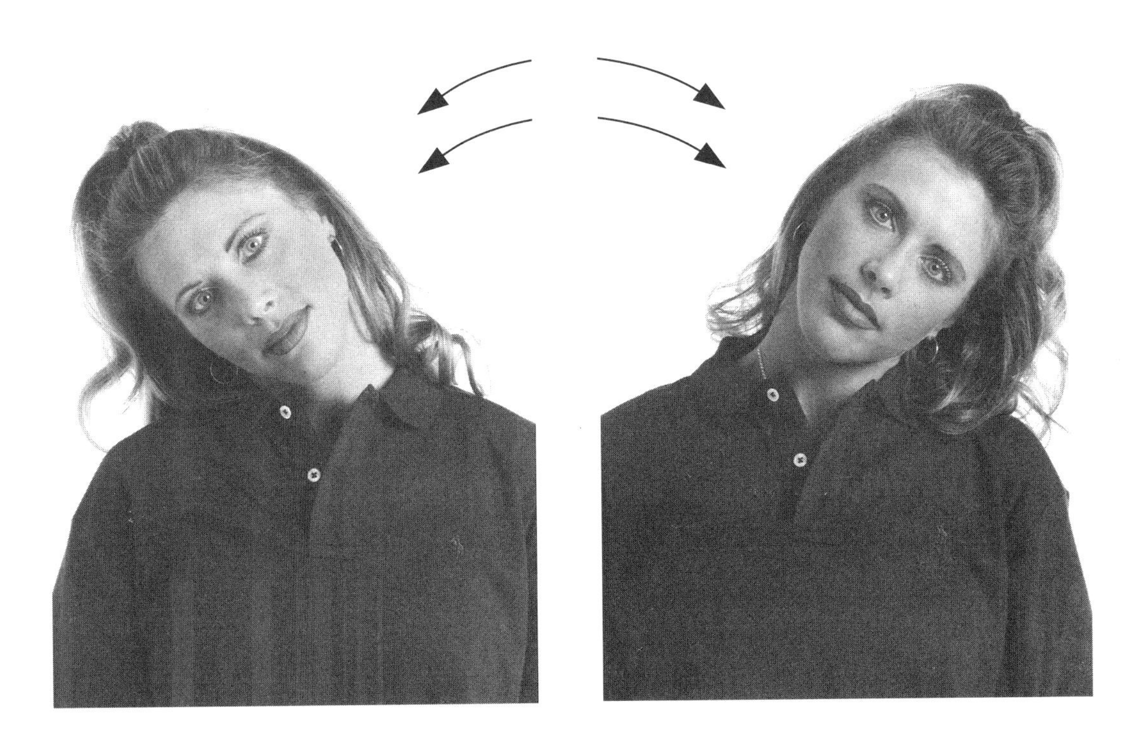

Simply stretch from side to side by lowering one ear toward the shoulder, then the other ear to the other shoulder. Hold in the stretch position for ten seconds and do ten repetitions for each side. Keep your shoulders lowered and relaxed throughout the exercise.

Neck stretches *(continued)*

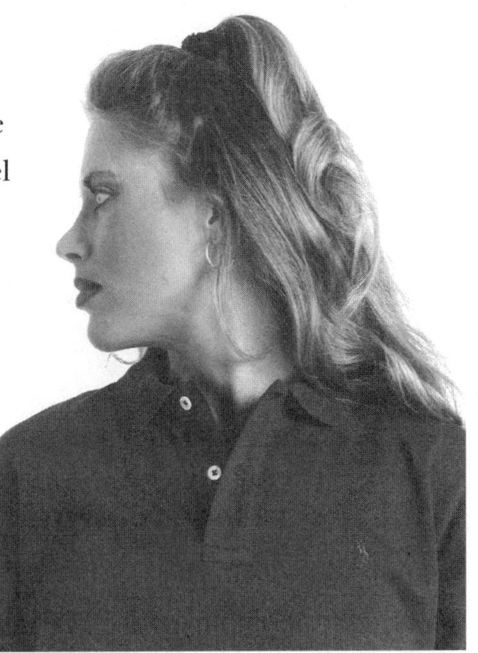

Keeping your eyes level to the ground, rotate your head back and to the right, until you feel a light stretch. Hold for ten seconds. Then rotate your head to the left and hold for ten seconds. Repeat ten times alternating to the left and the right.

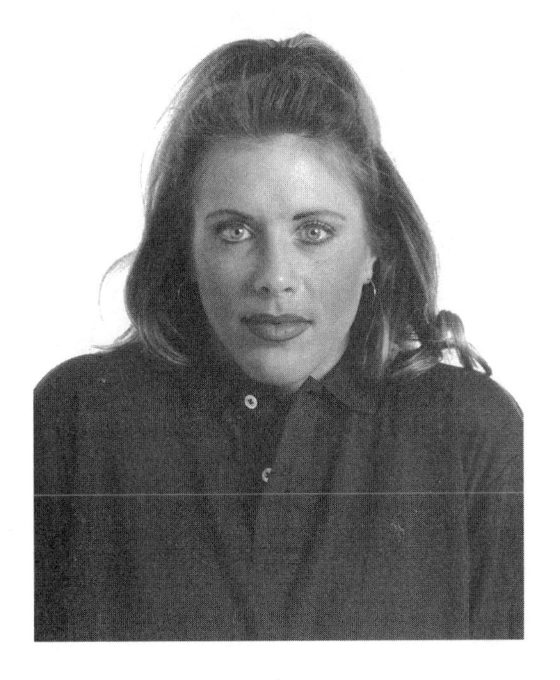

Shrug your shoulders, raising them toward your ears as high as they will go, and get rid of the tension. Hold for ten seconds, then release. Repeat ten times.

Exercises to do at work or at play

The following exercises are done standing up, at home, when at work, or anywhere outside.

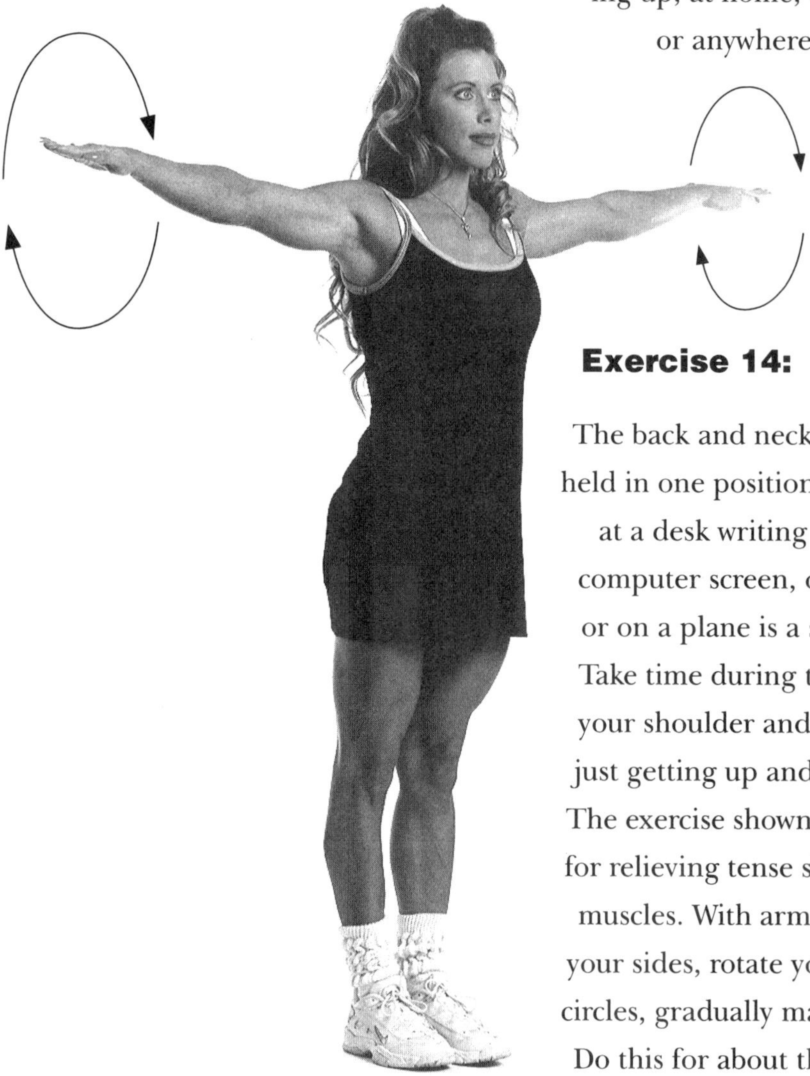

Exercise 14: Arm circles

The back and neck do not like being held in one position. Sitting for hours at a desk writing or looking at a computer screen, or sitting in a car or on a plane is a set-up for strain. Take time during the day to loosen your shoulder and neck muscles by just getting up and moving around. The exercise shown here is also good for relieving tense shoulder and back muscles. With arms outstretched to your sides, rotate your hands in wide circles, gradually making them larger. Do this for about thirty seconds at a time, then relax for a minute. Repeat several times, but don't strain.

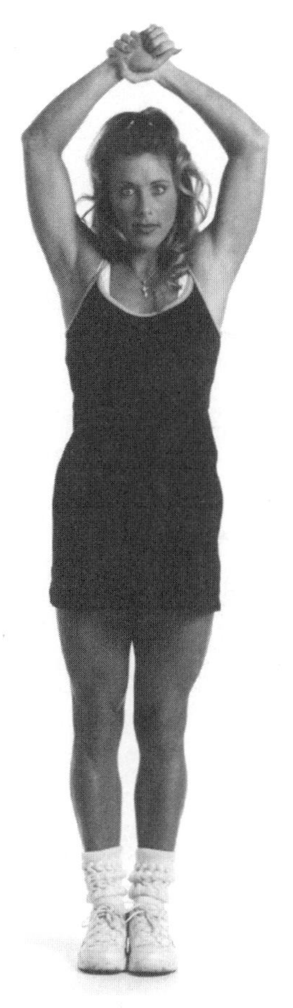

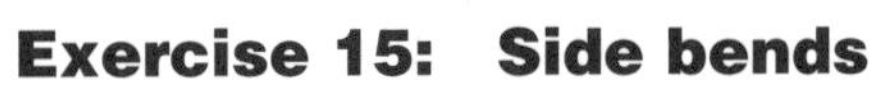

Exercise 15: Side bends

This is a great exercise to do as a warm-up for tennis, golf, or any other sport. With your hands overhead, wrist clasped, lean first to one side, hold for five seconds, then lean toward the other side and hold for five seconds. Repeat ten times. You should feel a gentle stretching sensation from your shoulders down to your lower back.

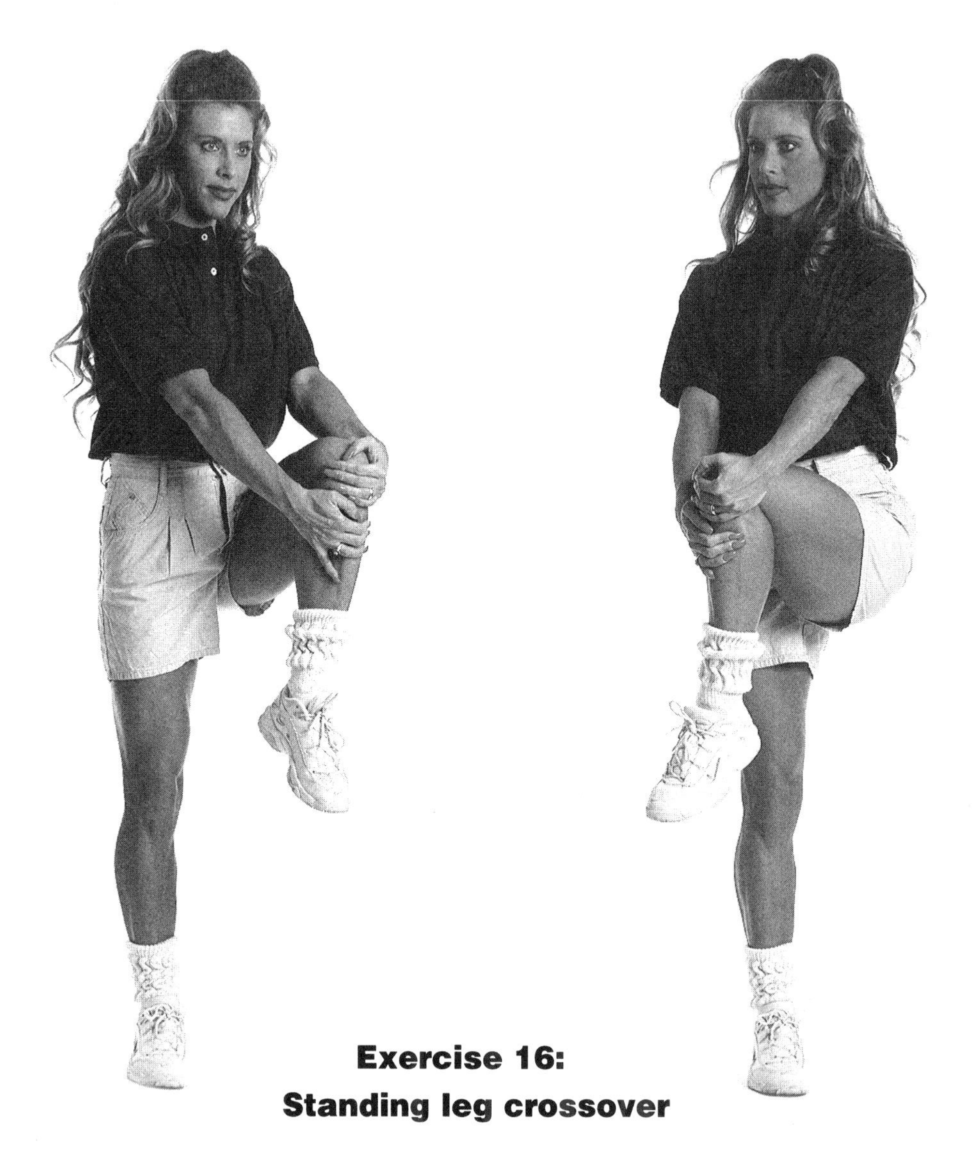

Exercise 16:
Standing leg crossover

You will see plenty of professional golfers with back problems doing this exercise throughout their round. On the first tee, or anytime your back starts to bother you during the day, stand and raise one knee into your hands, then cross the knee across your trunk. To help with balance, lean against a wall or a tree. Hold the stretch position for ten seconds and then repeat with the other leg. Do ten repetitions of this stretch.

Exercise 17: Standing lumbar rotation

Rotational sports really test the spine. Anyone getting ready for a rotational sport like racquetball, tennis, or golf should warm up with this exercise. Otherwise, an abrupt coiling could cause an unpleasant strain. Put a golf club, tennis racquet, or even a broom handle behind your neck and rotate from side to side, holding each stretch position for five seconds. For golfers, simulate the rotation of the golf swing by bending over slightly at the waist while you rotate.

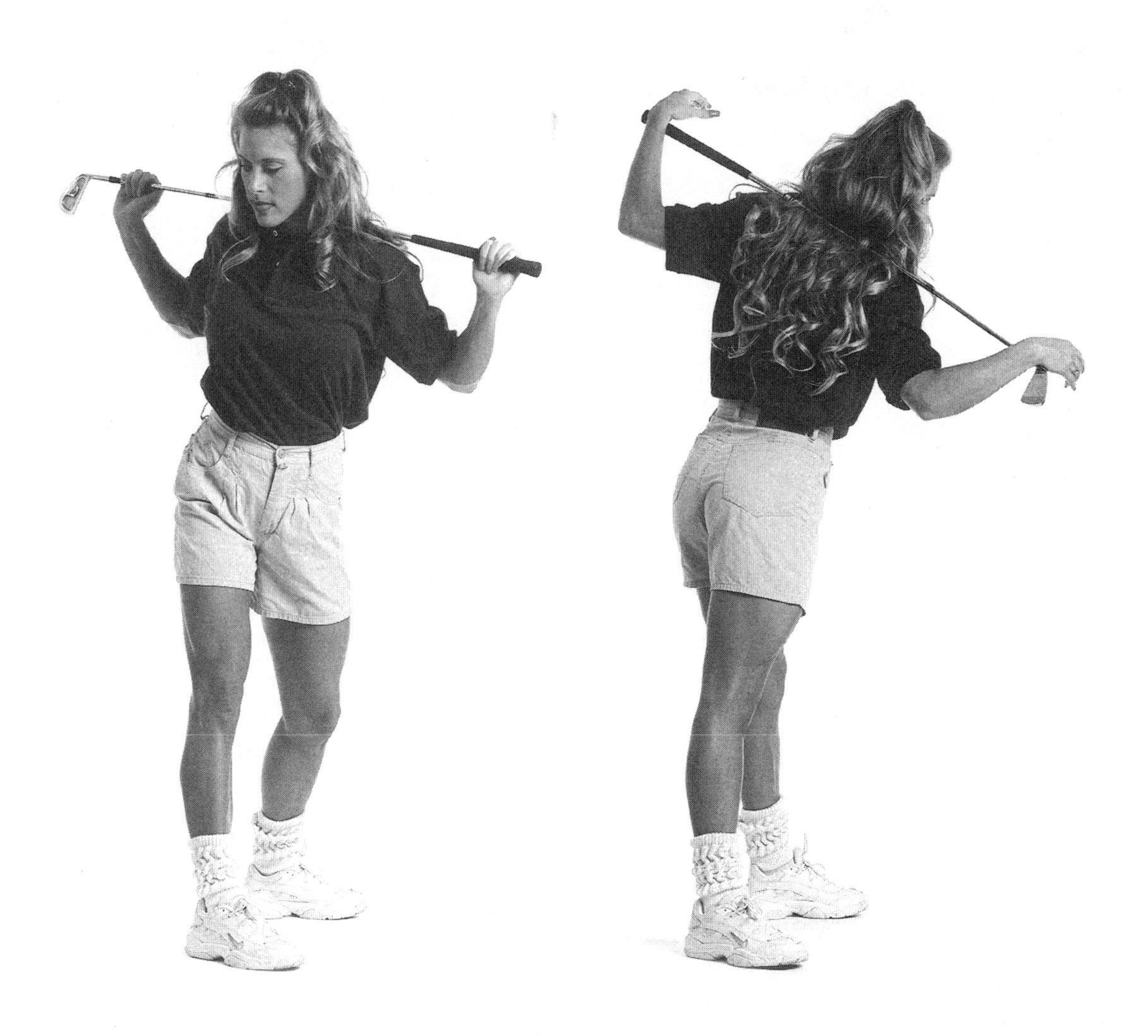

CHAPTER 4

Mainstream Professional Remedies

In 1986, the *New England Journal of Medicine* published a somewhat ground-breaking paper that ended the long-held belief that back pain should be treated with inactivity and bed rest. The researchers found that for most back pain, bed rest should be limited to two days at most. Then the patient should be encouraged to get back to activity.

Even the way physical therapists have treated back and neck pain has been revamped over the last 10 years. It used to be common for a back pain patient to lie on a table and wait for a therapist to apply ice packs, hot packs, ultrasound devices, and other passive "modalities."

Now, physical therapists who are experts at back pain treatment use these modalities very little. The physical therapists who have advanced spine training are proficient in special McKenzie exercises, hydrotherapy, manual therapy techniques (similar to the principles involved in chiropractic), and other special bending and stretching movements that slowly and gently increase the flexibility of the tender muscles and ligaments in the back. Professional remedies also include injections and chiropractic manipulation to achieve pain relief.

Physical therapy

Physical therapy is perhaps the most mainstream of all non-surgical cures for back and neck pain. When a patient has excruciating back or neck pain, it is the role of the physical therapist to provide some pain relief. Physical therapy can also relieve pain, correct poor body movement patterns such as your gait, improve posture through stabilization exercises, and strengthen the muscles that support the spine.

Physical therapy falls into two categories: passive and active.

The passive pain-relieving techniques used by a physical therapist in working with back or neck pain are called "modalities." A passive pain-relieving modality — where the therapist is doing something to you — is only a means to an end, however. Ultimately, your long term rehab program will involve exercise, where you are playing an active rather than a passive role.

As part of your treatment with modalities, the therapist may apply heat packs or ice packs to your back or neck. The function of ice is to restrict circulation to the injured tissues and reduce inflammation. Typically, ice is used for the first 48 hours after an injury. Later, heat may be used to increase circulation and encourage the flow of oxygenated blood, which will help heal sore tissues. The therapist may also use ultrasound, which sends heat deeper into muscle tissues.

A physical therapist may also use electrical stimulation, called transcutaneous electrical nerve stimulation (TENS), to relieve pain. In this procedure electrodes are taped to the body and a mild electric current is applied, which helps to relieve pain symptoms.

Therapeutic massage is another modality that can feel good when recovering from back pain, provided the person giving the massage is professionally trained. Rough or untrained massage on a sore back is not helpful and could cause more problems if you have a herniated disc. Never let anyone — not your friend, spouse, Aunt Mildred, or Uncle Harry — do any manipulation of your back or neck unless they are a licensed chiropractor, osteopath, or physical therapist.

Lastly, some progressive therapists are learning manipulative therapy techniques, which resemble chiropractic manipulation. This use of manipulation by therapists illustrates how far spine care has come in the last 10 years. In the 1980s, physical therapists and chiropractors viewed each other with disdain. Then in the early 1990s, the more advanced chiropractors began providing therapy and exercises as part of their care plans. Similarly, in the last few years, more spine therapists have learned manipulative therapy techniques to help patients get moving quicker. Interestingly, the lines between all the disciplines are beginning to blur.

All these modalities are pain-relieving techniques designed to help the patient move to the next step: active exercise. It is only when the patient begins these exercises that the sore muscles begin to regain their flexibility and strength. Consequently, it is important to view the most constructive part of your therapy as the point when you start doing things for yourself, not when the therapist is doing things to you.

In this regard managed care organizations have influenced the care patterns of both therapists and chiropractors, by putting pressure on both disciplines to accelerate patient recovery. Generally, managed care organizations discourage an emphasis on physical therapy modalities. They don't want to pay for massages, hot packs, and ice packs. If they are paying the bill, they want to see the back or neck pain sufferer moving quickly into more productive supervised exercise.

Typically, the better the spine clinic, the less the emphasis on modalities. Sure, everyone would like a back rub and a heating pad, but research has shown these don't rehabilitate the back strain. So you should expect your spine therapist to try to wean you of these modalities as soon as possible. As soon as you can tolerate it, your therapist will begin moving you toward the therapy gym within the clinic, to get you into special exercises that stretch out the sore muscles and increase their flexibility.

As you move along in treatment in the rehab gym, you will work with a variety of personnel. Your exercise therapy may be done with an exercise physiologist — an expert in exercise — or an athletic trainer. An occupational therapist may also be involved. This expert can help you learn how to do specific job-related activities in ways that don't strain the back. For example, if you are a carpenter your occupational therapist may show you how to lift and carry a ladder or a large plywood board in a way that doesn't strain your back.

As you move closer to recovery, your physical therapist or exercise physiologist should design a home exercise program that is geared for your specific back problem. Just like a dentist who will evangelize you to always floss your teeth after meals, your therapist will stress that you need to do your back exercises every night — for the rest of your life. Consider it preventive maintenance.

Group back schools and other back education

If you go to a back specialty clinic, your doctor may prescribe that you attend the clinic's back school. A back school is a group class that lasts anywhere from one to four hours, and is typically conducted by a physical therapist. The program will often cover the anatomy of the spine, so you get a better understanding of how you hurt yourself and what you need to do to recover from strain. Wear comfortable clothes to the back education class, because the instructor may get attendees involved in performing floor exercises to relieve back pain and strengthen sore muscles. You will also learn the correct way to lift objects and perform daily activities so that you don't strain your back again.

Group back schools are nothing new, in fact, they have been around for more than 15 years. The Texas Back Institute was one of the first specialty centers to offer group classes to patients. Over the years, the group back school has gone in and out of fashion. Recently, the idea of a group class about back anatomy and how to prevent back pain is coming back in vogue as hospitals reinvent themselves as community wellness centers.

Do group back schools work? Some Swedish studies show that those people who attend back schools learn lifting skills that prevent a future back strain. Other research, however, has not demonstrated a strong correlation between back schools and lowered risk of future back pain attacks.

Part of the problem was that, in the past, some clinics herded large groups of adult patients into a room and let a physical therapist lecture them on anatomy for two hours. The setting had the effect of group anesthesia, and many adults would tune out and take a nap.

Many clinics now believe that it is more effective to have a therapist work one-on-one with patients, educating them in proper lifting techniques. Where the instruction must be done in groups, the therapist may involve the class in lifting exercises to provide interaction and improve retention. So, depending upon where you go, a clinic's back school may be a one-on-one, intensive program with an occupational therapist or physical therapist, or a group class, or both.

A 1997 study in the Scandinavian *Journal of Rehabilitation Medicine* found that a functional restoration program that involved back pain sufferers for a three-week intensive program using work simulation and back education had superior results in getting people back to work, helping them stay physically active, and reducing their dependence on pain medicine, compared to more brief back schools or physical training.

Generally speaking, most back experts believe in the benefit of people learning how to lift, push, and pull in ways that won't strain the back in the future. It is logical that knowledge is beneficial, especially when it can prevent a future problem. How that education is provided is what will determine if people benefit from the training. As with any subject, group education may not be as effective as one-on-one training.

Chiropractic

Chiropractic developed in 1895 with a focus on the body's ability to heal itself. The original ideas gave a significant role to the nervous system in maintaining the balance of bodily function. Problems in the joints, particularly of the spine, were thought to interfere with the nervous system, upsetting the balance of body functions and causing symptoms. Modern chiropractic recognizes that muscles, bones, and joints are important in maintaining functional balance. Chiropractors attempt to restore normal function and relieve symptoms through the use of manipulation of the spine and other joints and muscles. Treatment is often reinforced by patient education, home exercise programs, rehabilitation, and nutritional consultation, where appropriate.

Although chiropractic has often been categorized as alternative medicine, it has gained broad acceptance. That is why we have chosen to include it here under mainstream cures instead of in the following chapter on alternative medical cures for back pain.

Some market research and recent scientific studies have shown that as many as 40 percent of back pain sufferers seek a chiropractor's services at some time for relief of back or neck pain.[1,2] So, if you use the level of public acceptance as a reference, chiropractic may be considered very mainstream.

While a large number of back and neck pain sufferers swear by chiropractic, some M.D.s are unsure about it. Part of the problem is that we do not have a full understanding of how chiropractic works. At the same time, credible scientific research on it has appeared over the past two decades and continues to become better known. The process of adopting new approaches in medicine seems to move slowly. This has the benefit, however, of allowing for as thorough a review of clinical benefits as possible.

One thing is clear: for whatever reason, and however it works, there are a lot of people who feel that chiropractic helps their back pain, and recent evidence supports it as a method worth trying.

The U.S. Government in the mid-1990s gave a significant endorsement when the Agency for Health Care Policy and Research (AHCPR) formally recommended that for back pain of less than three months duration, simple exercise, over-the-counter medication, and spinal manipulation were preferable to extended bed rest, prescription painkillers, and surgery.

At the same time, chiropractic is *not* an end in itself. Most modern Doctors of Chiropractic augment their manipulation of the spine with exercises that strengthen the back and make it more flexible, stronger, and resistant to future strain.

Chiropractic still needs to build bridges to managed care despite evidence that, used appropriately, it can be cost effective.[3] There are a growing number of managed care plans that offer direct access to specialists including chiropractors. However, other plans still restrict appointments with chiropractors unless the patient has a prescription from a primary care M.D., which may be tough to get since some M.D.s don't believe in chiropractic.

At the most progressive back institutes across the nation, the lines between all back care providers are blurring. Physical therapists are learning more about manipulating the spine, and chiropractors are incorporating exercise physiologists in their practices. Orthopedic surgeons are doing neck surgeries which were once the exclusive domain of neurosurgeons. Neurosurgeons, similarly, are learning to use instrumentation to stabilize the spine, which was once the exclusive domain of orthopedic surgeons.

In some cases, both orthopedic surgeons and neurosurgeons are working closely with Physical Medicine and Rehabilitation (PMR) specialists who argue against surgery altogether. All of which can

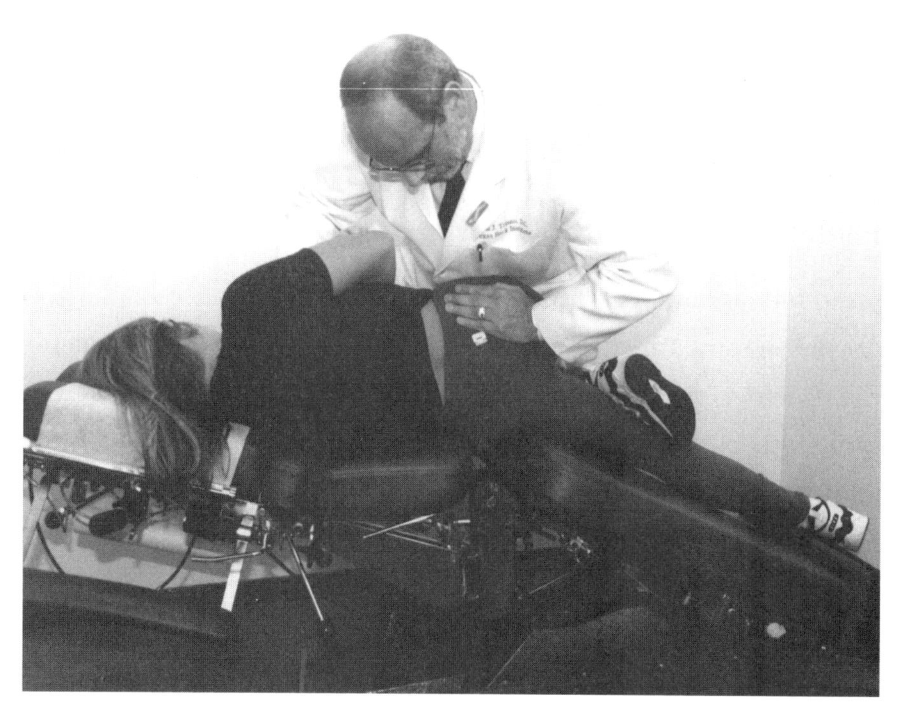

The U.S. Government's Agency for Health Care Policy and Research (AHCPR) has endorsed chiropractic for relief of simple back pain. (Photo courtesy of the Texas Back Institute)

make for some interesting physician meetings at the end of the day when doctors discuss their cases. But the real benefit of this blended approach is to the consumer, who gets the best of all possible kinds of care.

All forms of treatment have some degree of risk. With manipulation of the spine, the scientific evidence shows that the risk of potential injury is extremely small and quite comparable to that of safe medical procedures. Chiropractic has been practiced quite actively in the United States and in over 80 countries.[4] While there are some problems that get great play in the media, like the herniation of a disc in the lower back, or paralysis from neck manipulation, these events are rare. According to the editorial director of the American Chiropractic Association's web page, Chiropractic OnLine, there is a greater risk of getting hurt in a car accident on the way to a chiropractor's office than from any treatment given by the chiropractor. There have been fewer than 35 cases of disc herniation of the lower back reported in the literature since the 1930s.[5] For serious complications following neck manipulation, clinical scientists have estimated the risk at about 1 in 1 million.[6]

Many managed care plans view chiropractic as safe and as a treatment that has fewer potential side effects than receiving too many drugs, injections, or an unnecessary surgery.

Injections

For years, spine physicians have used cortisone injections, epidural steroid injections, trigger point injections, and nerve blocks to relieve pain in the spine. These injections are really intended as a means to an end. The theory is that by injecting pain-relieving medication directly into the site of injury or the pain generator, a patient can make the transition from inactivity to the physical therapy gym. Once there and able to move, the patient is ready for physical therapists to begin to work their wonders.

Spine injections are often provided in a series of three or four injections given over a couple of weeks. The theory is that a series works better at knocking down pain and inflammation than a single shot.

There has been some conflicting research about the value of various injections. Some studies have questioned the benefit of epidural steroid injections. Another authority, Britain's Royal College of General Practitioners, noted in their back care guidelines released in 1997 that epidural steroid injections relieve lower back pain with sciatica (leg pain) better than some other treatments. The Royal College is less supportive of facet joint injections and trigger point injections, however. According to them, there is little supporting evidence that these injections improve clinical outcomes.

Many spine specialty centers believe in the benefit of injections and continue to use them. Some experts theorize that there may be a placebo effect associated with the relief that accompanies an injection. In any event, when a patient gains relief after an injection, it reinforces a physician's desire to use that treatment again. As with many treatments, spine injections probably need more study before a definitive conclusion can be reached about their benefits.

Lumbar corsets, traction, braces, etc.

Decades ago, people with simple back pain attacks would end up in traction on a hospital bed. That is now ancient medicine for back pain. The same is true for lumbar corsets, braces, and anything that attempts to put the back into a state of traction or immobility. Britain's Royal College of General Practitioners, noted in their 1997 back care guidelines that lumbar corsets and supports have not been proven to reduce back pain.

Notes

1. Carey, T.S., Evans, A., Hadler, N., Kalsbeek, W., McLaughlin, C., Fryer, J. "Care-seeking Among Individuals with Chronic Low Back Pain." *Spine* 20 no. 3 (1995): 312–317.
2. Carey, T.S., Garrett, J., Jackman, A., McLaughlin, C., Fryer, J., Smucker, D.R. "The Outcomes and Costs of Care for Acute Low Back Pain Among Patients Seen by Primary Care Practitioners, Chiropractors, and Orthopedic Surgeons. The North Carolina Pain Project." *New England Journal of Medicine* 333 no. 14 (1995): 913–917.
3. Mosley, C.D., Cohen L.G., Arnold, R.M. "Cost-effectiveness of Chiropractic Care in a Managed Care Setting." *The American Journal of Managed Care* (1996): 285–292.
4. *WFC Report*. World Federation of Chiropractic, Toronto, Ontario, Canada, November 1997.
5. Haldeman, S., Rubenstein, S.M. "Cauda Equina Syndrome in Patients Undergoing Manipulation of the Lumbar Spine." *Spine* 17 no. 12 (1992): 1469–1473.
6. McGregor, M., Haldeman, S., Kohlbeck, F.J. "Vertebrobasilar Compromise Associated with the Cervical Manipulation." *Topics in Clinical Chiropractic* 2 no. 3 (1995): 63–73.

CHAPTER 5

Non-Surgical Cures from Around the World

When you were little and felt sick, remember how good it felt when your Mom knelt down in front of you and gave you a big hug?

What does a hug have to do with back or neck pain? A lot, apparently. If you have exhausted the traditional approaches to relieve your back or neck pain, if needles and drugs and physical therapy have left you frustrated and still in pain, you may want to enter the world of alternative medicine. But before you enter this world, you need to know the keys to success: faith, and an open mind.

If you enter as a skeptic, turn around and go back. It is not worth your time. To get the most out of your exploration of this world of alternate medicine, you must open your mind to believe that things you don't understand may actually work. For example, how can you explain why a hug can comfort you or make you feel better? Is there some surge of well-being that comes from it? Is it endorphins? Did Mom clear your energy pathway?

Science can't say for sure. Some skeptics argue that relief may be due to a placebo effect, that is, some people will get better because they convince themselves that the treatment they are receiving should work.

Modern medicine has made dramatic leaps forward in technology over the last 30 years. But consider this: some of the techniques described in this chapter date back thousands of years. Acupuncture goes back to at least 100 B.C. in ancient China. If it were completely without benefit, don't you think it would have been abandoned centuries ago?

In our own nation, consider the medical practices within American Indian tribes. Did you know that many of the herbs and tree roots that American Indians collected and used to treat various medical problems at least 200 years ago contain the same biochemical agents as some of the drugs commonly found in today's medicine cabinets?

While we as Americans are more comfortable with the concept of how chemicals and surgery can alter our bodies, when exploring the world of alternative medicine we should consider that in our bodies there might be unexplainable and invisible energy pathways that regulate our health thermostat and control how fast we recover from injury. Imagine that these energy pathways are like a complex freeway system with interlocking roads and crossovers. An injury may upset things, causing a blockage. Using a mind-body technique, magnets, or herbs might correct the energy flow and restore health.

If you suffer from chronic pain, you know that most medical doctors are stumped by your condition. They either can't explain why you hurt, or they may be at a loss for effective treatments. It may be time to explore a different world of medicine.

Some physicians are quick to disparage alternative medicine and things that have no scientific explanation. What does managed care think about it? You'd be surprised. A 1997 survey of 300 executives of health maintenance organizations (HMOs) reported that nearly three-fourths of HMO professionals believe spirituality can reduce health care costs. The same portion of HMO executives believes God or some higher power can sometimes influence recovery. On the other hand, 90 percent of health plans currently disregard the link between spirituality and health. While the HMO executives intuitively believe spirituality may influence care, they add that they would need to see studies that show it saves money and improves patient satisfaction. Studies involving alternative medicine and mind/body healing will surely be hot over the next decade.

The fact is for now, much of alternative medicine is unexplainable. So recognize that your hard-line medical doctor may criticize some of the approaches in this chapter.

But what do you really have to lose? The alternative medicine treatments discussed in this chapter are probably worthwhile things to explore before you resort to surgery, and for the most part they have few of the downsides that surgery does.

Alternative medicine advocates say that too much emphasis is placed on surgery, drugs, and other high-tech diagnostics and treatments in the mainstream treatment of back pain. They believe the body is better served through a holistic approach to diagnosis and treatment that includes the mind (spirit, intellect, and emotion) and the body (organs and tissues).

While recognizing the significant achievements of modern medicine, this "mind-body" approach is based on the belief that health can only exist when both mind and body work in balance with one another and in harmony with the body's own natural rhythms and cycles.

Some of the treatments discussed in this chapter date back as far as 5,000 years. Also, keep in mind that some things Americans view as "alternative medicine" are widely accepted and practiced throughout the world.

The traditional medical establishment in the United States has recently begun to test and experiment with alternative treatments. An increasing number of studies are beginning to document results from alternative medicine. For example, a 1993 study published in the *New England Journal of Medicine* revealed that alternative medicine is now a $10 billion industry. The study noted that one in three Americans regularly uses some form of alternative health care.

The people who are choosing to use alternative medicine might surprise you. One study out of Harvard Medical School found that it was mostly highly-educated baby boomers, some very wealthy, who were likely to try alternative medicine. As healthcare consumers, they are fed up with paying high fees for an impersonal 15-minute exam by a traditional doctor. They note that an alternative medicine practitioner will often spend an hour with the patient on a first appointment, asking personal questions about their problem and their emotions. Not surprisingly, more of a bond is created between patient and healer.

In 1992, Congress directed the National Institutes of Health to conduct research and create an Office of Alternative Medicine. These researchers are now studying acupuncture, herbal medicine, and biofeedback. The National Institutes of Health's Office of Alternative Medicine (OAM) operates an informative web site with a frequently asked questions (FAQs) section and subsections on various health problems and alternative medicine solutions. The site can be accessed at http://altmed.od.nih.gov/oam.

Some advocates of alternative medicine argue that conventional medicine looks at physical causes and sometimes overlooks non-physical causes. Chronic conditions, they argue, are often caused by multiple factors, which supports the argument for taking a more holistic approach. Plenty of people would benefit from new techniques that provide relief from chronic conditions. For instance, the *Journal of the American Medical Association* reports that about 100 million Americans suffer from chronic disorders such as heart disease, high blood pressure, asthma, and arthritis.

Natural medicine takes into account preventive measures as well as the body's own healing mechanisms. The Arthritis Foundation observes that more arthritis sufferers are exploring acupuncture, a Chinese technique discussed below that is based on using tiny needles to restore the body's energy balance.

Some managed care companies are keeping an open mind on the issue as well. Chiropractic can be a covered benefit under certain plans, and even acupuncture is starting to be covered by some plans. In some cases, managed care organizations are realizing that alternative medicine treatments can be much less expensive than traditional medical treatments like surgery.

The alternative medicine treatments discussed in this chapter are a sampling of the techniques that are more widely available in this country and have some proven success in the treatment of back pain.

Healing with touch

The power of touch is not well understood, but more people involved in healing are starting to return to using touch as part of what heals us. Traditional M.D.s are extremely poor in the art of touch. Many of them, as if by training in medical school, avoid touching the patient. One of the things that sets chiropractors apart from M.D.s in their treatment approach to back pain is that a chiropractor touches the patient a great deal in the process of spinal manipulation. Conversely, the M.D. typically only touches the patient during the first physical exam. Thereafter, the physician performs medical management with a prescription pad or a needle. That is changing, however. Some medical schools are training new doctors to connect better with their patients.

Biofeedback

If the concept of a mind-body link to your health sounds far-fetched, consider that medical science has extensively embraced the beneficial effects of biofeedback, in which the person regulates their pain level through their thought process.

Biofeedback is probably one of the more scientific means of exploring the mind-body connection. Through the use of electrodes placed on the body, biofeedback attempts to measure a physiological function, convert this measurement into an understandable form, and then feed back this information to the individual.

The electrodes detect the body's physiological responses to pain by measuring body temperatures, heart rate, muscle tension, skin resistance, and perspiration. When placed on muscle groups, the electrodes record changes in their electrical activity. The needle on the biofeedback machine indicates contractions (high electrical output) and relaxation (low electrical output). The degree of response of the needle simply provides the therapist with a numerical measurement for muscle tension.

Advocates of biofeedback claim it enables the back pain sufferer to control and manage pain levels. There are two schools of thought about how this is done. The first believes that the back can be relaxed by focusing on one muscle group, while the second believes that it is possible to focus on total body relaxation, thereby reducing pain. Biofeedback can help "train" a back pain sufferer to avoid movements such as tensing of muscles and awkward posture to eventually eliminate pain.

Biofeedback therapists are licensed by the Association for Applied Psychophysiology and Biofeedback (AAPB). The AAPB can be reached at 800-477-8892.

Using metals and magnets

Have you been to a golf tournament recently? If not, watch closely the next time you see a golf tournament on TV. Look at the wrists of the pro golfers and even the caddies. Many of them wear copper wristbands that are supposed to relieve pain from sore tendons, muscles, and ligaments, or joint pain from arthritis. The theory is that the power of the mineral in the band filters into the body to relieve pain.

There are also several champion pro golfers who use magnets and swear that their golf games were saved by wearing metal discs on their backs. The discs are held in place by velcro belts.

These flat magnets are said to operate on the premise that the magnet has healing powers when applied on the body. Some doctors theorize that magnets help increase blood flow, and the increased oxygen-carrying capacity in turn enables the body to heal itself. Other theories maintain that magnets influence calcium ions which can heal bones more quickly, or migrate calcium away from arthritic joints. Another premise of magnetic healing is that the body's normal pH (acid/alkaline) balance is thrown out of whack when the body is injured or sick, and magnetic fields help to restore that balance.

Body work

Body work is an umbrella term for the many manual therapy techniques used to promote relaxation and treat ailments through massage, lessons in proper movement, changing posture, exercise, and other body manipulation. Some types of body work such as massage can be practiced at home, others require a trained professional.

Advocates argue that by manipulating and massaging the body's tissues, and making changes to body posture, there is an impact on the body's circulatory, nervous, and musculoskeletal systems. The following sections describe specific areas of body work. There is a great variation in cost depending upon the type of body work performed. Some states regulate massage therapists with registration or licensure. Call your state's Board of Health, Department of Health, or State Board of Medical Examiners for a list of qualified treatment providers in various areas, or to determine what certifications may be needed in your state.

Massage Massage includes an assortment of techniques used to manipulate the soft tissues of the body to reduce tension and stress, increase circulation, aid in the healing of muscle and other soft tissue injuries, control pain, and promote overall well-being. Massage is believed by some to do the following:

- trigger the release of endorphins
- increase blood flow
- reduce inflammation
- remove tension and cramps from muscles
- stimulate the circulation of immune system cells
- break down scar tissue
- calm the nervous system

Swedish massage is the most popular form in the United States. Developed more than 150 years ago, the technique involves five key strokes. *Effleurage* helps the therapist to learn the subject's body through the use of stroking motions extending from the neck to the base of the spine and from the shoulder to the fingertips. *Petrissage* increases circulation, and attempts to clear out toxins from muscle and nerve tissue by gently lifting muscles and tissue from the bone and gently massaging them. *Friction* breaks down muscle "knots" by applying deep, circular movements near joints and other bony areas such as the sides of the spine with the thumbs and fingertips. *Tapotement* releases tension and relieves muscle cramps by applying short, chopping strokes with the side of the hand, closed fist, or tips of the fingers. *Vibration* increases circulation by pressing the hands on the back or limbs and shaking rapidly for a few seconds.

Reflexology Reflexology involves manipulating or applying pressure to certain areas of the feet or hands that correspond with organs in the body to eliminate energy blockages that may produce pain and disease. Practitioners of reflexology claim it can relieve a wide variety of ailments.

Feldenkrais Method Feldenkrais method involves movements and stretches that make you more aware of your posture as you stand, sit, walk, or bend. In short, the method tries to retrain your muscles to avoid positions that may cause pain and discomfort.

The Alexander Technique The Alexander Technique is based on the belief that posture, specifically the alignment of the head, neck, and spine, can affect back and neck disorders. Advocates of the technique feel that back strain can be reduced by improving how patients balance their body weight on their spines while standing, sitting, and walking. Generally speaking, the goal of the Alexander Technique is to allow the spine to lengthen in the way one stands, sits, walks, and stretches. The technique was created by a performer who discovered that certain changes in posture improved vocal performance, and it may take 30 sessions to learn. Not surprisingly, the technique continues to be popular with singers and stage performers.

The American Center for the Alexander Technique in New York City was the first center in the nation focusing on the technique. Some physical therapists around the country have incorporated the Alexander Technique into their treatments. Some of the principles are similar to standard physical therapy treatments that focus on helping the patient stabilize the spine through specific postures.

Rolfing Rolfing is a deep tissue massage technique developed by Dr. Ida Rolf. It involves penetrating massage and vigorous movement to loosen or release adhesions in the connective tissue covering the muscle in an attempt to bring the body into correct alignment. Actually, Dr. Rolf had a strong background in yoga before she invented Rolfing. She died in the late 1970s, but her technique is still practiced in many specialty massage centers.

The premise behind Rolfing is that over time we develop specific body movements that accommodate our physical misalignments and pain symptoms. A hip injury or leg strain may have caused us to shift our weight distribution or change our gait to reduce pain. In turn, the connective tissue in our bodies stretches and adapts to these particular postures. The long term result is that this connective tissue can bind us into these unbalanced postures and movements. In some cases connective tissue may shorten on one side of our bodies, pulling us further out of balance. Dr. Rolf believed that if this connective tissue could be loosened, it could give the person a fresh start at achieving a balanced and proper posture and gait.

For example, the Rolfer may detect that the person has slipped out of proper vertical alignment, letting the head slump too far forward. Through the use of deep massage techniques, the Rolfer works to release the body's tension and get joints and ligaments moving freely. The Rolfing technique can reportedly be quite painful, especially to someone already suffering from strain. Still, there are those with back pain who swear by the benefits brought by Rolfing.

The Rolf Institute, which trains Rolfers around the country, is based in Boulder, Colorado.

Aston Patterning Judith Aston graduated from UCLA with degrees in dance and fine arts. In 1967, her life changed after a couple of car accidents left her with back pain. According to her doctors, her dance career was over. She experimented with a variety of therapies before finding dramatic pain relief in a Rolfing session. Subsequently, she collaborated with Ida Rolf to develop an entire movement program that incorporates Rolfing techniques.

Aston Patterning is a technique that imparts correct posture according to the particular characteristics of each person's body. Aston believes that each body is unique and needs its own proper method of movement. She believes that our bodies are somewhat elastic and, over time, people begin to mold their posture to their environment, such as slumping down into the chairs in their home or office. Aston Patterning attempts to break that negative mold.

The Aston Training Center is located in Mill Valley, California.

Chinese medicine

If you are biased toward mainstream American medicine, consider that American medicine dates back only a couple of hundred years while Chinese medicine goes back thousands of years. In recent years there has been a growing similarity between the medicine practiced in China and the United States. Chinese doctors use the same high-tech diagnostic equipment as doctors in the United States. In turn, American M.D.s are looking more closely at Chinese medical techniques that have been used for centuries. Both cultures are seeing benefit in each other's approach to healing.

Chinese medicine is one of the most intriguing types of medicine. Considering that its evolution has been very separate from that of Western medicine, there are many similarities in how we treat and evaluate problems. There are also interesting differences that are worth studying.

The traditional Chinese doctor's exam — called the Four Examinations — may include inquiring, looking, listening/smelling, and touching. The intent is to identify patterns of disharmony of essential substances, organ systems, and channels. The doctor might examine your tongue, facial color, voice, smell, pulse, and sensitivity to touch.

Chinese medical treatment could involve acupuncture and moxibustion, acupressure, or herbal medicine. The term herbal medicine is slightly misleading, however, as the medicines may be derived from plants or animals.

Acupuncture Traditional acupuncture is based on the ancient Chinese theory that there are energy pathways that run throughout the body. These pathways, called meridians, carry the body's vital force or energy, called *chi* (pronounced "chee"). It is believed that there are 14 meridians — 12 bilateral and 2 unilateral. The principle behind acupuncture is that disease and pain are caused by the body's energy flow (chi) being out of balance.

Through the insertion of thin needles at specific points along the meridians the flow of energy is controlled and rebalanced in the body. Usually five to fifteen needles are inserted at specific points anywhere from a fraction of an inch to four inches deep.

Acupuncture dates back in China to the first century B.C., during the era of the Han dynasty (206 B.C.–220 A.D.). Chinese medicine sees all disease processes as disturbances in the flow of energy through these meridians and related internal organs. Because Western physicians in the United States have difficulty understanding the correlation between acupuncture philosophies and traditional physiology, acupuncture has not been accepted readily in the United States.

Acupuncture is used to treat a variety of ailments, including back pain, joint pain, digestive disorders, general aches and pains, sinus problems, headaches, stress, and anxiety. Ideally, acupuncturists hope for permanent relief of symptoms. Sometimes symptoms can resurface and a few more sessions may be needed to gain relief.

Compared to physical therapy and other traditional Western treatments, acupuncture is reasonably priced. As with traditional medicine, the first visit is more expensive, but probably less than $100. In most major cities, the cost for traditional acupuncture sessions ranges from $35 to $75 per treatment.

Researchers over the years have tried to learn why acupuncture appears to relieve pain. They have performed dissections of cadavers to see if there is a correlation between the Chinese meridians and nerve pathways. A 1977 study claimed to show a 71 percent correlation between trigger points — the specific area of a muscle that is spasming — and acupuncture points. Another study showed a high correlation between acupuncture points and muscle motor points.[1]

Contrary to what you might think, in most cases acupuncture causes little pain, with the exception of a tiny prick that may be felt when the needle first enters the skin. Some describe the sensation as similar to a mosquito bite, others say they don't feel anything. It does not feel like an injection with a hypodermic, for instance.

The needles used by an acupuncturist do not resemble the needles we are used to seeing on the end of a syringe. By comparison, acupuncture needles are flexible and some may be about as thin as a human hair. Unlike hypodermic needles which are hollow to allow for the injection of a liquid, acupuncture needles are not hollow because nothing is injected through them. They also have tapered tips.

Once the needles are inserted, you may feel warmth or a tingling sensation. If you have pain, the needle may appear to make the pain go away. Some find the sensation relaxing.

Some people feel an immediate effect while, others may need seven or eight sessions before they experience pain relief.

An acupuncturist may also perform a treatment called moxibustion, where the heat from smoldering herbs is applied directly just above each acupuncture point.

Several studies have documented the effectiveness of acupuncture in relieving pain in laboratory animals. There appears to be some evidence that acupuncture stimulates the release of endorphins and other neurotransmitters which serve as natural painkillers. But scientific research still remains unclear on how acupuncture provides long-term pain relief.

The practice of acupuncture is licensed in 26 states. In 1991, the U.S. Surgeon General endorsed the World Health Organization's plan to prepare guidelines on training, safety, regulation, and research in acupuncture. In 1992, the National Institutes of Health created the Office of Alternative Medicine. Grants for research in acupuncture have been included in the budget since 1993.

Acupuncture, pardon the pun, got a shot in the arm in early 1997 when the U.S. Food & Drug Administration (FDA) approved acupuncture needles as legitimate medical devices. Earlier, the FDA had classified the needles as investigational. The effect of the change is that now, according to the U.S. Government, acupuncture needles are classified as safe to use, and the Health Care Financing Administration and Medicare could begin steps to recognize their use as a covered procedure.

In late 1997 a National Institutes of Health panel concluded after an exhaustive literature review and scientific presentations that acupuncture can reduce nausea caused by surgery, chemotherapy, or pregnancy. It also is effective in relieving pain after dental surgery.

Acupuncture is also gaining mainstream credibility among more traditional allopathic M.D.s. There is now an American Academy of Medical Acupuncturists with 1,000 M.D. and D.O. physician members.

In southern California, the University of California at Los Angeles (UCLA), a prestigious medical mecca, conducts a special course in acupuncture for physicians through its Office of Continuing Education at the UCLA School of Medicine. While many such continuing education courses for physicians take 30 hours, the medical acupuncture course takes 200 hours for doctors to complete. More than 1,000 physicians in the United States have completed the course.

The practice of acupuncture has not been limited to China. European physicians, especially doctors in France, have used acupuncture since World War II. Acupuncture, over time, has become a standard part of medical school training in France.[2] In 1980 an estimated 6,000 physicians in France were routinely using acupuncture in their daily practice.

Electro-acupuncture Some physicians have adapted traditional acupuncture techniques. Since the 1950s, for instance, Chinese physicians have applied a low voltage electric current to acupuncture needles for different pain management techniques. There are two basic approaches. One approach uses low-frequency but high-intensity current. This procedure is believed to produce pain relief that is slow in onset, is more generalized throughout the body, and continues after the electrical stimulation stops.

The second approach uses high-frequency/low-intensity electric current. This produces pain relief that is rapid at onset, is more related to the specific location of the needle, and typically stops when the electrical stimulation stops.

Another key difference is that the first approach may tend to produce a cumulative pain relief effect, where the second approach does not.

Acupuncture advocates stress that for acupuncture to work, you must have a series of treatments, one after another, that build up such a cumulative pain relief effect.

Craig PENS acupuncture One technique, called Craig PENS (Percutaneous Electrical Nerve Stimulation), involves attaching electrodes to acupuncture needles. Electric current is then transmitted through these needles into the body.

The key difference between traditional acupuncture and the Craig-PENS technique is that needles are placed more in line with spinal nerves rather than traditional meridians. Interestingly, though, the meridians that relate to the back closely mirror the pathway of sciatic nerves that branch off from the spine and travel down the leg. Consequently, for lower back pain that travels down the leg, the physician may place needle electrodes in the lower back and down the leg along the path of the spinal nerve. The electrical current is maintained at various intensity levels for about 20 minutes. A few days later, the patient will return for another session. For successful treatment, a patient should have about 10 to 15 sessions to notice improvement.

The use of electrical stimulation on spinal nerves has a lot in common with spinal cord stimulators, which are also covered in this book, although spinal cord stimulators are more commonly used as a last-ditch treatment for people whose back surgery didn't work.

By directing electrical current through strategically placed acupuncture needles, the physician is attempting to stimulate the peripheral nerves and nerve roots. The theory behind the procedure is that neurotransmitters involved in transmitting pain signals maintain a delicate balance between suppressing pain and transmitting pain. When this balance is upset because of tissue damage or inflammation from injury, the balance may shift in favor of the neurotransmitters that transmit pain signals rather than suppress pain signals.

Under this theory, chronic pain is a failure of these transmitters to regulate themselves correctly. The use of electrical current and the acupuncture needles is believed to play a role in restoring this delicate balance.

Does it work? The ultimate goal, according to Dr. Stephen Taylor of Fort Worth who uses the technique on his patients, is to provide pain relief that could last up to a year or more. Dr. Taylor notes that he has suffered from chronic back pain since being diagnosed with a herniated disc at the L 4/5 level at age 23. Over 25 years of living with his back problem, he has at times been limited to walking with a cane. In 1994, he underwent 20 sessions with the Craig-PENS procedure.

Nine months later he was hiking in the mountains with a 50-pound backpack. Now, at age 48, he confides that he has some lasting numbness in the leg from the herniated disc, but thanks to the Craig-PENS treatment he no longer suffers from the incapacitating, searing radicular pain that used to travel down into his legs.

While an ultimate goal may be pain relief that lasts a year or more, more frequently the Craig-PENS technique appears to help some patients reduce their pain for at least few days.

Two patients interviewed while undergoing Craig-PENS at Dr. Taylor's clinic confided that their pain first got worse after four or five sessions, as anticipated, but then improved following several more sessions.

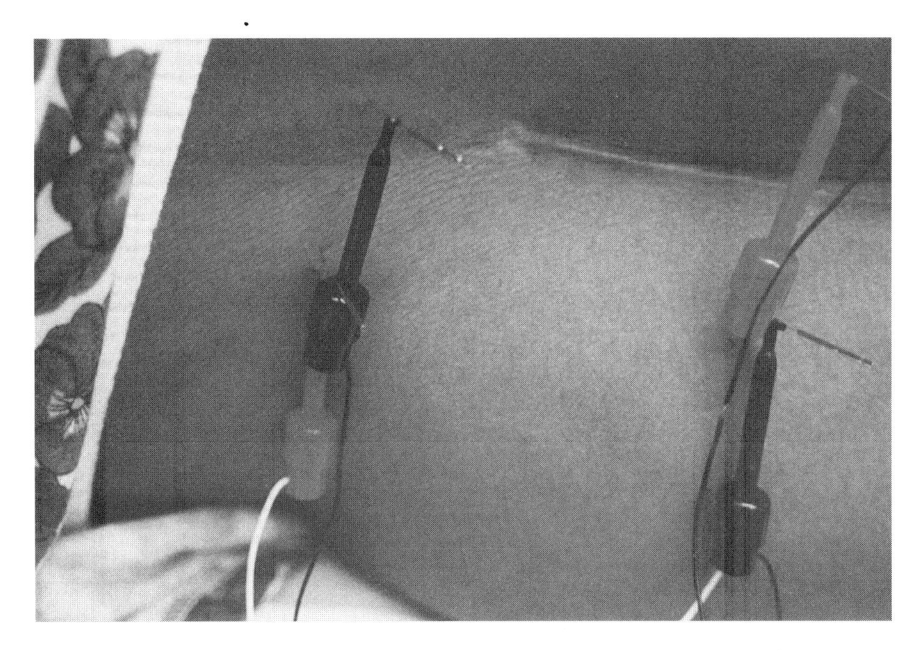

A patient's scar from unsuccessful lower back surgery is visible as she receives Craig PENS acupuncure for pain relief.

One patient who had a back injury from a car accident had back surgery but was worse afterward. She tried injections, drugs, and physical therapy to reduce the pain all without success. She entered Dr. Taylor's clinic in a wheelchair and now is able to walk short distances. More importantly, she has reduced her dependence on heavy drugs. Before starting the Craig-PENS treatment she was taking more than 10 pills a day for relief of pain and had difficulty sleeping through the pain. Now, with the acupuncture technique helping to reduce the pain, she is down to three pills a day and can sleep better.

The second patient noted that she had also exhausted traditional treatments of injections and physical therapy and had not obtained relief from a stabbing pain that ran across her lower back and down her right leg. She now finds that an acupuncture session provides complete pain relief for several days.

Dr. Taylor notes that the long-term goal is to find ways to make the procedure's pain-relieving effects more long-lasting. Even if the pain relief is temporary, it still is a worthwhile alternative to expensive injections or heavy dependence on drugs.

Ear acupuncture One of the more amazing aspects of acupuncture is that sometimes the acupuncture point that treats a certain pain complaint is located away from the part of the body where the pain is.

For example, some cases of back pain can be treated with needles that are inserted into the external ear cartilage. After the needles are removed magnets or even seeds may be applied on the acupuncture point for further stimulation.

If treating the ear for back pain or anxiety sounds farfetched, consider that the ear is one of the first things to form during fetal development, along with the brain and spinal cord. The ear may actually be hard-wired into our central nervous system.

Pain in one part of the body can often be caused by problems elsewhere. For instance, it makes perfect sense in Western medicine to treat pain that radiates into the leg by addressing the source of the problem — a disc in the lower back.

The bottom line on acupuncture Between 1976 and 1989 there were 14 controlled studies on acupuncture for treatment of lower back pain. Seven of the studies concluded that acupuncture was better than no treatment, TENS, and trigger point injections. Several of the remaining studies were not so favorable when comparing acupuncture to TENS or injections, though some studies were found to be flawed in their execution.[3]

Like many holistic remedies, research still needs to be done to help medical practitioners understand how and why something works or doesn't work.

Modern science has taken a shot at explaining how acupuncture can relieve pain. Some observe that the traditional Chinese "meridians" overlap with some of the pathways of the central nervous system. By using needles, the acupuncturist can stimulate the nervous system to release endorphins (morphine-like chemicals) in the muscles, spinal cord, and brain. These chemicals either relieve the pain symptoms, or trigger other chain reactions that relieve pain symptoms.

Because acupuncture is non-surgical, doesn't involve drugs and the chemical dependency that may result, has no real negative side effects, no permanent complications, and is relatively inexpensive compared to more expensive options, it may be worth exploring when you have exhausted the traditional remedies of Western medicine. Some states regulate acupuncture through licensure. Ask if your acupuncturist is "licensed." Some Chinese physicians may use M.D. after their name if they have a medical degree from China, or O.M.D., which stands for Oriental Medical Doctor. There is also the National Certification Commission for Acupuncture and Oriental Medicine that is involved with certification of acupuncturists based on exams and testing. The commission can be reached at 202-232-1404. They may be able to provide you with a list of credentialed acupuncturists in your area.

Acupressure If you are squeamish about needles, consider acupressure, which is based on the principles of acupuncture. Acupressure involves changing the flow of energy by applying pressure with just the hands or fingers and thumbs on the same points used in acupuncture. A single point may be pressed or multiple points may be worked in a specific order as needed.

It is difficult to learn acupressure effectively from a book, as the skill requires an in-depth knowledge of the meridians or energy pathways. The best approach for self-care and to fully appreciate the potential of acupressure is to locate a therapist who can train you in working on the specific acupressure points that can relieve your specific pain symptoms.

According to Chinese medicine, sciatic pain that radiates from the lower back into the leg is caused by a disruption in the flow of energy (chi) through the energy channel meridian that travels from the liver/kidney area down into the leg. By using acupressure to stimulate a blockage point along this meridian the energy flow along this pathway can be restored, much like using a tow truck to remove a car wreck that is clogging an expressway during rush hour traffic.

Tai chi Hundreds of years ago, tai chi (pronounced "tie chee") was a closely guarded secret in ancient China, taught only to a select few. It is believed to date from the 13th century, and was originated by a Chinese monk. Gradually it became more widely known and the basic movements were used by the Chinese as a healing exercise.

The most common forms of tai chi practiced in the United States today involve extremely slow and precise arm and leg movements, resembling the scripted ritualistic martial arts movements from the same culture. But unlike martial arts, most tai chi involves no impact or jarring movements, which makes it excellent for older people. In addition to the stretching movements of various parts of the body, a 20-minute tai chi exercise session promotes deep breathing, and the constant shifting of weight from one leg to the other develops good balance skills, all of which can make for a good workout and stress release. For advanced practitioners there are also other forms of tai chi that involve quicker hand and leg movements and more challenging postures that stress the legs.

It is estimated that during the 1950s in China up to 200 million Chinese used tai chi exercises daily. More recently, in the United States, the National Institute on Aging sponsored a study that was published in the May, 1996 issue of *The Journal of the American Geriatrics Society*. The study took 215 people over the age of 70 and split them into three groups. One group received weekly tai chi lessons, one group worked on balance exercises, and a third group worked on behavior modification to see if balance and agility could be improved. The researchers found that within the group of seniors using tai chi, blood pressure decreased, grip strength increased, and the participants noted they felt more in control of their lives. A year and a half later, the tai chi group had reduced their risk of falling by one-half, the only group of the three studied to decrease this risk.

Advocates of tai chi argue that the exercises have wide benefits. Some women claim that the exercises reduce cramping associated with menstruation. Other proponents say the exercises relieve stress, improve posture, and can actually relieve back pain and other musculo-skeletal symptoms.

As it relates to the back, some spine specialists advocate tai chi for patients because it emphasizes postural stances and balance that can assist a person with back pain. It enables the person to relax, which helps muscles regain flexibility. The exercises also encourage the participant to breathe deeply, which reduces tension and back pain. Through deep, focused breathing, paying attention to the painful area, pain can exit the body.

To get a feel for Tai Chi, try these simple exercises:

1. **"Fill the balloon":** Start by sitting in a chair. Place one hand on your chest and the other hand on your stomach. Observe your breathing closely. Feel which hand moves as you inhale and exhale. Breathing from the chest restricts circulation to the body, and when circulation is inhibited, muscles get tense and pain increases. Strive to feel your stomach move, as if you are filling a balloon when you inhale.

2. **"Riding a Horse":** Sit in a comfortable chair with your back relaxed. Lower your chin toward your chest so the weight of

your head falls forward. Now lower your left shoulder, collapsing your left side and allowing your head to roll toward the left. Let your right shoulder rise and your right side stretch and open up. Repeat for the other side, rolling your head toward the right, collapsing your right side and stretching out your left. Do this several times, rolling your head back and forth, gently stretching your sides and releasing the tension in your neck.

Qi gong Qi Gong (pronounced "chi kung") is an ancient Chinese discipline emphasizing breathing, meditation, and exercises to increase one's internal energy and keep it flowing freely throughout the body. Some experts believe that the art was originally brought to China by an Indian Buddhist. Qi stand for energy and Gong means achievement.

One can begin to understand the principle of Qi Gong by watching children at play, witnessing how they immerse themselves fully in the enjoyment of the present moment. What may come naturally to children, however, may take some work for adults. Check you local martial arts or tai chi studio for lessons in Qi Gong.

In Qi Gong exercises, if you focus your mind on your lower back, the energy flow will be directed there and healing will begin. This may be similar to how acupuncture works. Consider what happens when a needle is placed in your lower back: you think about it, you focus on it, and perhaps the energy flow is directed there by virtue of your mind.

In a sense, Qi Gong exercises are similar to yoga, tai chi, and other "slow" movement exercises. There are exercise poses where you move, sit, or stand. Not all are easy. Some exercises or poses can require the patience and mental strength of a Buddhist monk. However, they can be helpful to get a person moving again and focused away from tension and toward relaxation.

Pain relief from India

Ayurvedic medicine Ayurveda (pronounced "ah-yur-vay-da") means "knowledge of life" and dates back 5,000 years in India. Ayurvedic theory suggests that all diseases stem from stresses in the awareness or consciousness of the individual. These stresses lead to unhealthy lifestyles which, in turn, produce a cycle of bad health. More simply put, disease, pain, and ill health can all be linked to being stressed out, which can make sense.

There are three stages to recovery. The first is *panchakarma*, which involves detoxifying the body of impurities and toxins by means of enema, vomiting, yoga, meditation, or chanting. During *tonification* (enhancement) the patient eats certain herbs and does breathing exercises and yoga. The third step, *satvajaya*, attempts to reduce emotional stress and release negative feelings through meditation. Ayurvedic medicine also uses dietary planning and herbal supplements to reduce pain. Many people will recall the fascination with transcendental meditation during the 1970s. Meditation, a key component of ayurvedic medicine, has been shown by the American Heart Association to lower blood pressure.

Ayurvedic medicine is believed by some to help those with back pain, neck pain, arthritis, Parkinson's disease, headaches, and asthma. A lot of emphasis is placed on prevention. Some herbs used by practitioners have been found by the National Cancer Institute to inhibit the growth of cancer cells.

Ayurvedic medicine is receiving more prominence from celebrity doctors like Deepak Chopra, M.D., a well-published author on mind-body healing, who also left his chief of staff position at a hospital to travel the country conducting seminars and book tours promoting the benefits of ayurvedic medicine.

A visit to a practitioner of ayurvedic medicine is not cheap, and can range up to $200. Some programs can last several weeks and cost thousands of dollars, which has led some critics to claim that some people are profiting from its popularity.

Yoga Yoga emphasizes strength, balance, flexibility, and spinal alignment through gentle, gradual exercises combined with meditation. While yoga can be great for stress reduction, some of the positions may be too uncomfortable for someone suffering from back pain. There are some yoga instructors who gear their exercises to people suffering from back problems.

Interestingly, some of the most popular yoga positions are identical to some of the exercise positions shown in this book which are espoused by clinically trained physical therapists. For example, the list below has the yoga position name, and the corresponding physical therapy exercise we use in the exercise section of this book:

Yoga position	Exercise name	Found on page . . .
Cat	Lumbar flexion #6	p. 46
Cobra	Advanced press up #10	p. 50
Half Cobra	Extension #1 position 2	top of p. 41
Sphinx	Extension #1 position 3	bottom of p. 42

Knee down twist	Exercise #4	bottom of p. 44
Shoulder crunch	Neck exercise	bottom of p. 55

For those back pain sufferers who become active again through the above yoga positions illustrated in this book, and want to explore more yoga positions, contact the International Association of Yoga Therapists, located in Mill Valley, California, at 415-383-4587.

A final thought about alternative medicine

Remember: while alternative medicine has shown some benefits and has practitioners, believers, and advocates, it is important to start your quest for a non-surgical cure with a medical doctor to rule out any medical condition which could become life-threatening.

Then, if you have a green light, open your mind to all the possibilities held in the world of alternative medicine. Keep in mind that there are thousands of miracle recoveries where people recover from terminal illnesses and their recovery can't be explained by science. Some wish to let religion take credit. Others believe in special treatments, potions, or spells. Whatever the operating principle, it is fair to say there is a mind-body connection that is not well understood in Western medicine.

Notes

1. Helms, M.D., Joseph, M. *Acupuncture Energetics: A Clinical Approach for Physicians.* (Publishers Press, 1995).
2. ibid.
3. ibid.

CHAPTER 6

Preventing Back Pain

In terms of remedies, we saved the best for last — prevention. It is ironic that, while prevention is the best back pain remedy of all, it is one we never think of until after we get back pain. And that, unfortunately, sums up the sad state of healthcare in the United States. We gear all of our medical weapons of war toward illness treatment and damage control, instead of educating Americans to prevent the illness in the first place.

That's how breast cancer was dealt with 20 years ago — but not anymore. Over the past 20 years, doctors have educated women to check their breasts for lumps and to get regular mammograms so they can detect and treat cancer early, with removal of a small lump rather than a breast or, worse, having the cancer spread throughout the body.

Prostate and testicular cancers, likewise, are starting to get some attention because of the various celebrities who have driven the issue to the forefront. Prostate and testicular cancers can be considered the male equivalents of breast cancer. Like breast cancer, both prostate cancer and testicular cancer can be screened for easily. And like breast cancer, if you don't detect prostate and testicular cancers early the consequences can be grim.

Heart attack treatment has also changed radically. The American Heart Association has spent millions over the past 20 years on heart attacks — preventing them, that is. Thanks to the AHA, now everybody knows the importance of checking their cholesterol level, using a low-fat diet, and exercising regularly. And simple chest pain? That has all of us running off to the doctor for massive lifestyle modification.

Unfortunately, there is not enough emphasis on preventing back and neck pain. People often ignore pain signals from their back and neck, continue lifting incorrectly, and never do flexibility exercises, so over time the problem gets worse and a person has a "back attack."

Fact: Once you have your first "back pain attack" you are four times more likely to have a recurrence. For someone with back or neck pain, that is not an encouraging statistic.

The fact is, back and neck pain amounts to a big and expensive problem for employers, managed care organizations, health insurance companies and anyone else who has to cover the high cost of back surgery. It is the most expensive and prevalent of all on-the-job injuries and the second-leading cause of days off work behind the common cold.[1] One of every three on-the-job injuries is a back or neck injury.[2]

Most of the cost comes from time away from work. Disability payments to those off work suffering from back pain cost up to three times as much as the actual medical care.[3] While no one can be sure of the total bill, some peg the cost of back and neck pain at somewhere between $20 billion and $100 billion.

When you compare spine problems to other health problems, it is clear that no one is immune. Experts estimate, for instance, that 80% of Americans will have an attack of back pain at some point in their lives. Some researchers estimate that among working people age 18 to 55, as many as one in five may experience back symptoms in a given year. For people under 45, spine problems are the most common cause of disability. And forget about looking up your family history for risk of this health problem. Back and neck pain can come out of nowhere and strike anyone.

Are certain occupations high risk for back pain?

Back pain cuts across all occupations, but there are certain motions that are particularly hard on the back. Any motion that involves lifting and then twisting is risky. Not surprisingly, garbage collectors generate a high number of back injury claims. Nurses, similarly, are a high-risk occupation for back pain because their jobs involve moving heavy patients. Worse, it is difficult for them to get leverage or to use the power of their legs when trying to move a heavy patient from a gurney to a bed. Workers who lift and throw packages into trucks also do a lot of bending, lifting, and twisting, which can be tough on the back.

Labor intensive jobs aren't the only ones that stress the back, though. Ironically, the less you move with your back the greater your stress. For example, any job that requires you to stand in one place, or even sit in one place, for several hours — like along an assembly line — can cause back strain. If you work in such jobs, try to keep moving, or get up and stretch every 10 minutes. Some of the standing back and neck exercises shown in this book in Chapter 3 are easy to do at work and can be done in seconds or minutes.

If you like your job, chances are low that you will suffer a disabling spine injury. Some spine researchers have noted that people who don't like their jobs are more likely to have, or at least claim to have, a disabling work-related back injury. This is because, in many cases, if a person has a work-related back injury, he or she can collect disability payments from the employer's workers compensation insurance carrier for the time spent off work.

Depending upon which state they live in, and whether or not personal injury attorneys are involved, some back physicians may believe that spending a lot of time, energy, and money on a back pain patient may be a waste until the person's litigation has been resolved. Over the years, these physicians may have observed that those people who hurt themselves on the job often don't want to get better until their lawsuit or workers compensation claim has been resolved with their employer's insurance company.

Stress and job satisfaction

As we said earlier, if you lift heavy loads on the job, especially ones that require bending and twisting, you are at high risk for back pain. That's not surprising. But did you know job satisfaction is also one of the predictors of how quickly you return to work after a back injury? If you are self-employed, you are very likely to go back to work, mainly because if you are self-employed you have to work to eat. But if you work for an employer the picture is much more complicated. Psychological factors such as high occupational stress, anxiety, and depression have all been identified as risk factors for back pain.[4]

Depression

A very real side effect of chronic back and neck pain is depression, frustration, and irritability. These psychological side effects can in turn create hormonal responses that amplify the pain signals to the brain. This causes even more muscle tension, and further pain. A psychologist may be needed to provide a way to pull out of this self-defeating disability spiral. The psychologist can lead both group and individual therapy sessions to encourage patients to control the pain. One method is to encourage patients to find pastimes that can distract their minds from their pain.

Physical activity is promoted through paced activity schedules that are individualized to the patient. A pain psychologist is also necessary to help with the evaluation of pain patients. The goal of psychological pain assessment is to determine the contribution of affective, cognitive, and behavioral factors to the perception and treatment of pain. This evaluation can help in the formulation of reasonable treatment goals.

Some of the psychological symptoms observed are secondary to the pain complaint, while others may have been in existence before the pain occurred. Regardless of the chronological order, an adverse effect on the patient's response to treatment is likely to be observed if these psychological factors are not identified and treated.

Body build, breast size, and lifestyle issues

The extra weight from being obese or pregnant can affect the alignment of the spine, which can cause back strain. Some experts believe tall people sometimes have more back problems than others. Women with large breasts may also have some extra risk of back pain. Both tall people and women with large breasts may experience back pain because they subconsciously hunch their shoulders to appear less tall or to make their chests less prominent.

Lose extra weight Studies show Americans are getting more overweight. A government study by the Centers for Disease Control and Prevention covering the period 1988 through 1994 found that 34.8 percent of Americans ages 20 to 74 were overweight — a 9.4 percent increase over the previous period studied in 1980. The study used the standard Metropolitan Life Insurance Company height and weight tables which state that a 5' 10" man should weigh 165 pounds. How does weight correlate with back pain?

It is not unusual for a pregnant woman to experience lower back pain from the increase in weight and resulting strain on her lower back. Some physicians argue that overweight people are at similar risk for back strain.[5] There is some conflicting research, however, about whether obesity in itself "causes" back pain.

Overweight people may also have difficulty recovering from back pain attacks because of their overall deconditioning. Their recovery and rehabilitation may take longer than that of someone who is already in good shape. Many spine physicians will recommend to patients with back pain to stay fit and shed extra weight that will unnecessarily burden the back.

Quit smoking If you still smoke and need to hear it from someone else, here goes: quit smoking, it's bad for your back, too. Studies have shown that smokers have a risk of back pain 1.5 to 2.5 times that of non-smokers. Spine researchers theorize that smoking reduces the blood supply to the back, which may affect the elasticity of discs and encourage disc degeneration.[6] One study looked at identical twins, where one twin smoked and the other didn't. The smokers were found to have degenerative changes in the spine.

If you smoke, you may also have problems getting spine surgery if you need it. Texas Back Institute surgeons, for example, will often not perform fusion surgery until a smoker quits smoking because it can prevent a bone graft from fusing successfully. In other words, if you smoke, your surgical outcome will be affected negatively.

Posture and ergonomic issues

Lift, push, and pull safely As the exercises in this section demonstrate, it is always safer to push a large object than to pull it, because you can use your body weight when pushing. Also, when you pull, you place strain directly on your back.

When lifting, we recommend you use one of the two methods demonstrated here. In Method 2 you put one knee on the ground, pull the object up on your thigh close to your body, then stand up. Method 1 uses more of a squat and can place more strain on your knees as they flex upward when you stand. Never lift while bending at the waist. Always use the power of your thighs, which are extremely resistant to strain.

Lifting kids out of strollers or car seats are back strains waiting to happen. That's because children's tiny legs will invariably get tangled just as you are extricating them from the seat, all at the precise moment that your back is at peak strain. Try to lean in deeper and

Two good ways to lift and one way that is sure to wreak havoc

Lifting an object — Method 1

Squat with your knees apart and the object between your knees as close as possible to your body. Using your legs, stand up, bringing the object closer in to your body as you stand. Be sure to keep your back straight.

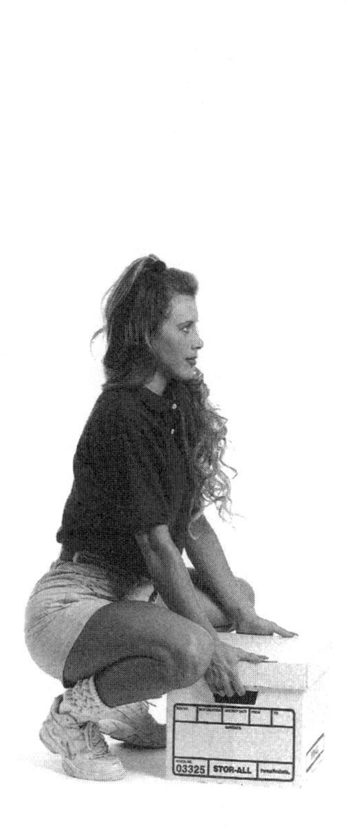

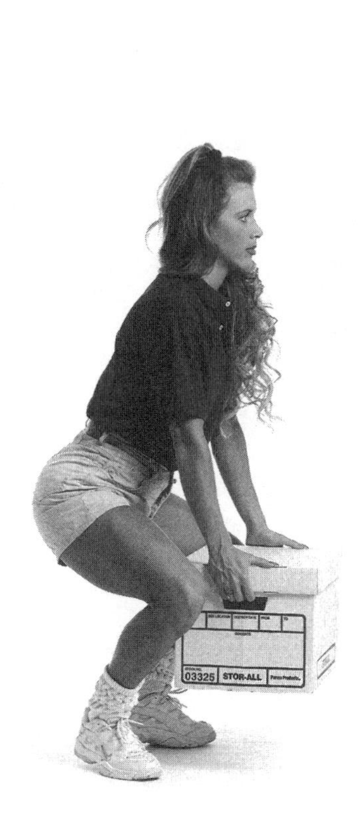

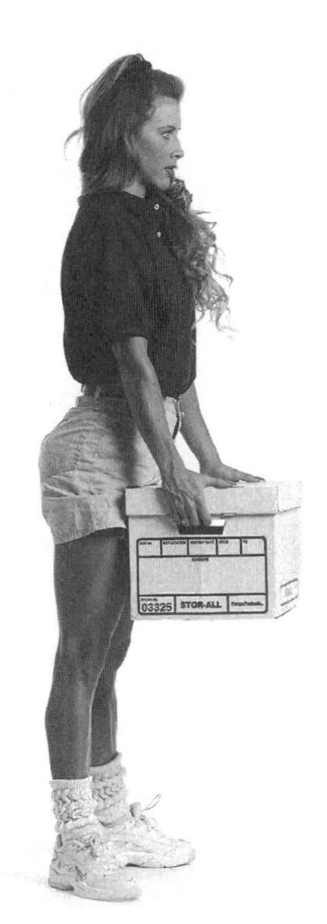

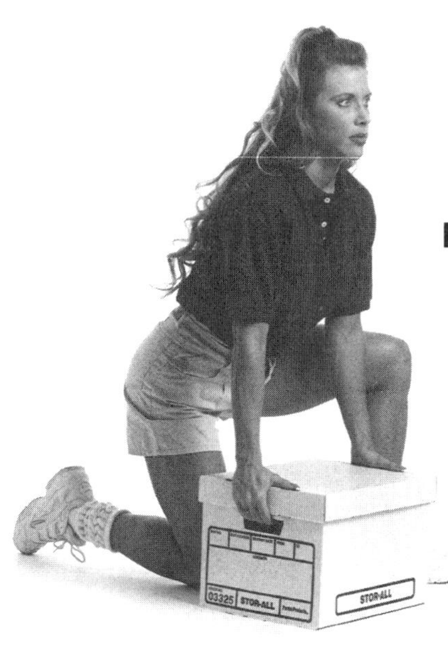

Lifting an object — Method 2

Put one knee on the ground. Using your arms, move the object uponto the opposite thigh. Then, simply stand up.

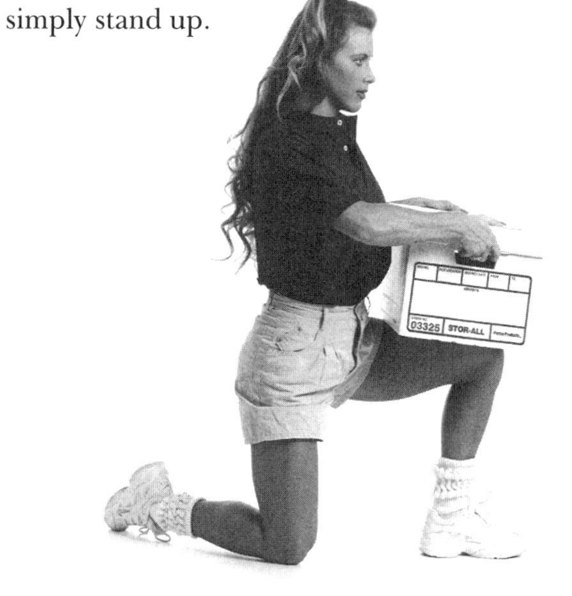

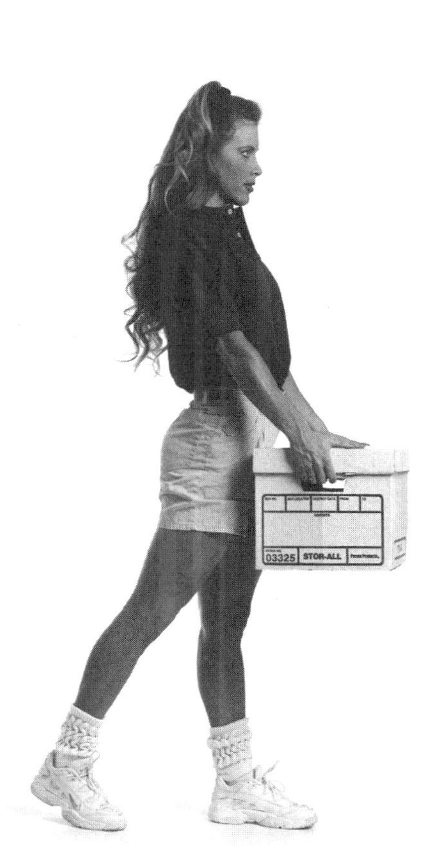

Photos by Paul Buck Photography, Dallas, Texas.
Photos courtesy of Prizm Development, Inc.

Never lift when bent over at the waist. This makes your lower back work like a crane, something it wasn't built to do. Always use the power of your legs to lift, not your back. Your legs are more resistant to strain.

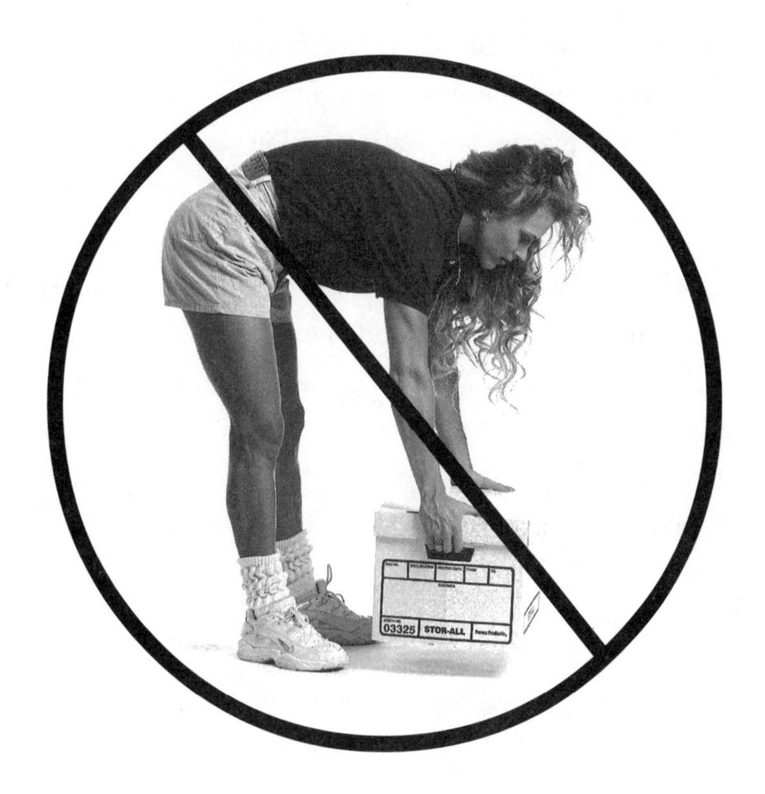

How to deal with really heavy objects: should you push or pull them?

When faced with a choice of having to push or pull something heavy, always push, never pull. Pulling will strain your back. By pushing, you can use all your body weight against the object. What if something is too heavy? Get help: a hand truck, dolly, wagon, or younger person to lift it.

place your knee on the car seat to get leverage. The same goes for lifting golf clubs and groceries out of a trunk, where you can't get the object close to your body. Place your knee on the bumper for leverage, and scoot the object over toward you before lifting it out.

How to stand for long periods You would think that standing is pretty basic, but standing for long periods of time can strain the back. For that matter, any static position that prevents the back from moving can be a source of strain. Secondly, because most people never really stand on two feet equally, the spine alignment can change. When standing, try to stand with your body weight balanced evenly on both feet. Another good standing position is to have a three-to-six-inch footrest. Stand with one foot up on the footrest for a minute or so, then switch legs. And give your back a break by using some of the standing back exercises from this book. Even taking only a minute here and there to let the back loosen up will lessen your risk of strain at the end of the day.

How to set up and sit at your desk Many employers who have paid out large amounts of money for back strain claims for employees have learned that sometimes it is a good investment to buy ergonomically designed chairs with good lower back support. In fact, most furniture manufacturers have redesigned their current products to provide a proper sitting position. If you have an older chair, consider buying a back support that rests against the back of your chair. Or take a rolled up towel and place that in the space between your lower back and the chair's back.

Once you have some lumbar support in your chair, the next step is to set the height so your feet are flat on the floor or resting on an inclined footrest. Your knees should fit easily under the desk, and you should be able to work without leaning or hunching over. If you type at a computer workstation, get one of the commonly available pads that enable you to rest your wrists at the keyboard. Your lower arms should be close to horizontal when your hands are resting on the keyboard.

The height of the monitor is the next item for adjustment. Some ergonomic designs actually sit the monitor into the desk below a glass pane, so the eyes only raise slightly to move from the keyboard to the monitor. Other experts recommend that the monitor sit more at eye level, raised up on a desktop computer, a special stand, or even a telephone book on top of the computer. But if you are a poor typist who has to constantly look back and forth between the keyboard and screen this can be a source of annoying neck movement.

Driving long distances Driving is another challenge for the back. Long-haul truck drivers, for example, are at high risk for back pain because the constant vibration of the road combines with the back having to hold a static position for long periods. If, at the end of the line, the driver then has to unload the cargo in the back of the truck, whammo, back pain.

As described in Chapter 2 about muscle anatomy, the piriformis muscle connects at the thigh bone and travels across the buttocks to the sacrum. The sciatic nerve, which extends into the leg, is affected when the piriformis muscle gets tight. Generally speaking, you are asking for trouble when you leave a muscle in a shortened position for a long time, as in a long drive. And if you drive with your knees apart, as most people do, this rotates the hips in a way that also negatively affects your piriformis muscle. On top of all that, sometimes men will have a fat wallet in their back pocket that sits right against the sciatic nerve, transmitting all the road vibration from the ground through the seat to the hard wallet, to the nerve. No surprise that, after a long trip, you go to unload the trunk and the first suitcase feels like dynamite going off in your back.

The best advice for driving is to stop often, get out of the car, and just walk around and do some stretches. Even a five minute stretch every hour will go a long way toward ensuring that your road trip has a happy ending.

Your neutral position If you have a bad back, one of the best investments you can make may be to get a customized home exercise program from a spine-specialized therapist. The therapist will educate you to find and maintain an ideal neutral posture in sitting and standing that takes the load off your back.

We are our own worst enemies when it comes to back pain. We stand in slumped over positions. We sit slumped forward or backward in our chairs at work. If you have a back that is predisposed to strain, you must fix your posture and find your neutral position.

Here's a quick way to check your posture and find your neutral position. Stand with your heels against a wall. Make sure your calves, buttocks, shoulders, and head are all touching the wall. Slide your hand behind the small of your back and shift your lower back to remove the excess gap. Step forward and see if your posture changes: it shouldn't. If it does, go back to the wall, recheck it, and step away. Learn this position and try to regain it as your neutral position.

If you sit at work, or spend a lot of time in the car, place a rolled up towel behind your lower back. If you stand a lot at work, change positions frequently. If possible, raise one foot on a foot rest, and change feet frequently. If you spend a lot of time sitting on airplanes, be sure to get up frequently and prowl the aisle. Sitting and vibration are bad combinations for the spine.

Corsets and back belts

If you've been to the gym lately, you may have seen some weight lifters at the squat rack lifting a heavy bar across their back to build up their legs. Many of these weight lifters wear a thick, eight-inch-wide leather belt across their back. Over the years, the concept has spread. Now you'll see luggage handlers at the airport wearing back belts as well. While the belt looks like it is supporting the back, the real theory behind the belt, technically speaking, is to increase the intra-abdominal pressure which in theory enables the person to lift more weight, over a longer period, without strain.

There is conflicting research on the subject of back belts. Proponents say they enable users to lift heavy loads without strain. Skeptics argue that this isn't proven. Both sides agree that wearing the belt does remind the user to be conscious of the risk of back injury, to lift using proper body mechanics, and not to lift something too heavy. In that sense, wearing a string around one's finger may accomplish the same thing. Those skeptical of back belts may argue that wearing a back belt may actually be a crutch, which may encourage some muscles to weaken, so that if the person has to lift when the belt isn't on there may be an increased risk of strain. The Texas Back Institute believes in belts but only when they are used along with exercise, not instead of exercise.

One research team looked at several popular ways commonly thought to prevent lower back pain. The group studied the use of back exercises; having people attend back schools where they learn how to lift, push, and pull with proper body mechanics; and the use of back supports, corsets, and back belts. They found that the best way to prevent lower back pain was through exercises that made the back stronger, more flexible, and resistant to muscle strain.[1]

Rotational sports

Tennis, golf, and racquetball are great for physical fitness, but be aware that these sports really place extra demands on the spine. Depending upon how moderate or severe your back problem is, you may not have to quit them, but you will have to warm up better and do exercises in the gym that strengthen the back muscles and obliques as well as increase their flexibility.

In tennis, the knees typically take the most abuse because of the running, lunging, and bending for volleys. The serve, however, does require some arch to the back. Depending upon your level of play, your professional can teach you a slice serve that requires less arching than a kick serve. Your choice of racquet may help your back. Typically, more flexible racquets (the kind most pros use) require longer, more fluid strokes to generate power. This type of stroke also requires more trunk rotation. A stiffer racquet with looser strings needs a shorter stroke to generate power. This can lessen the need for trunk rotation in the stroke. In summary, ask your pro about using a stiffer racquet strung at the lower end of the recommended string tension.

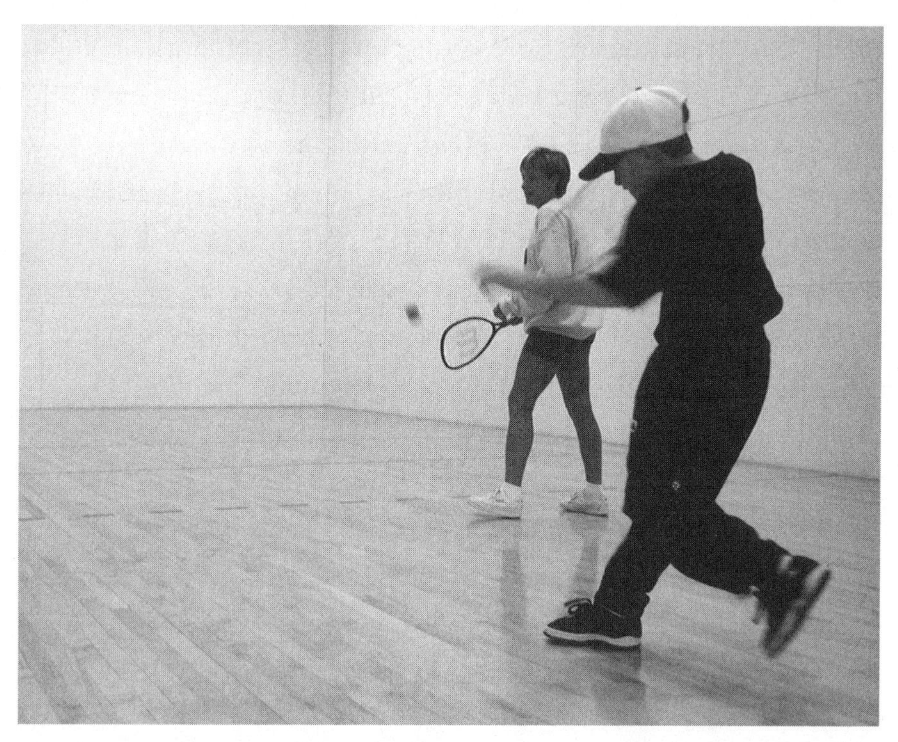

While most spine physicians will strive to get a person back to the sport they enjoy to encourage physical fitness, aggressive racquetball may be an exception. Because it requires a person to bend at the waist and rotate with great torque, racquetball may be too risky for someone with a disc-related back problem.

The Center for Spine in Savannah, Georgia, because of its proximity to the many beautiful Hilton Head golf courses, offers an instructional course conducted by a physical therapist and a local golf pro for golfers with bad backs. The therapist and golf pro work with golfers to improve their form, and teach them postures and techniques that lessen strain on the back. In some cases they recommend longer shafts on the shorter irons, like the 5-iron through wedge, that lessen the amount the golfer has to bend at the waist. Ironically, some back strains during golf come from something as simple as bending over and picking the ball out of the hole. This risk can be lessened by bending at the knees, or getting an adapter for the bottom of your putter grip that can pick the ball out of the hole without you bending over.

Racquetball is one sport that is especially hard on the back because it requires the spine to bend and twist violently. With racquetball, the objective is to keep the ball low on the front wall. The most effective "kill shots" are made by bending at the waist so you can strike the ball at its lowest point just above the court surface. This requires a player to bend at the waist, rotate the trunk, and sweep the ball with great wrist and trunk torque — a recipe for disaster. A person with a bad back may want to reconsider playing this sport, or at least play it less competitively.

High impact sports

Water skiing, snow skiing, dirt bike riding, horseback riding, and snowmobiling are examples of recreational activities that are extremely tough on the back. In addition to the jackhammer effect on the spine from constant vibration and jolts, all of the above activities also have risk of traumatic injury from a fall. Someone with an existing disc-related back problem should probably explore other ways of having fun.

Sleeping without strain

Researchers who measure the load placed on the spine in various positions have found that standing and sitting still require back muscles to do some stabilizing duty. Lying down is one of the rare times when the back muscles can take a break. Make sure, when you go to sleep, that you give your spine muscles a chance to completely unload their burden of your body weight. To do that you need to sleep properly. Sleeping on your stomach is the worst position for the back because it arches the back and twists you head to the side. No wonder people wake up with a stiff neck.

There are two ideal positions for sleeping. Lying on your back is excellent, and having a pillow underneath the backs of your knees is even better. Sleeping on your side is also an excellent position, especially if you can put a pillow between your knees. This helps to align your spine correctly.

Lastly, find a bed that is good for your back. In shopping for a mattress, or checking your current one, lie on your side and have a friend observe the alignment of your spine. Your spine shouldn't curve. If you have too soft a mattress the heaviest part of your body, your midsection, will sink in too far, which will curve your spine. A mattress that is too hard, on the other hand, may not allow your hips and shoulders to sink enough for a comfortable alignment.

Four ways to lower your risk of back or neck pain

1. Avoid falls, car accidents, and other traumatic injury. All it takes is a moment of distraction, maybe your car runs a red light or you trip down the stairs, and your life is changed forever.

2. You brush your teeth to prevent cavities. You avoid high fat foods to prevent a heart attack. What are you doing to prevent

back pain? You need to incorporate a regular series of home exercises, like those shown in this book, into your daily regimen. The easiest way to make time to work out is on your carpet when you are in front of the television. Put some of that time to good use.

3. Modify how you lift, using the proper body mechanics shown in this book. Also, remember you're not Hercules. The grim reality is that you may be 42, not 22, and you may need to get help to carry that 50 pound bag of fertilizer from the car to the garden. Or use your kid's wagon, rather than hauling it across the yard on your back.

4. Don't sleep on your stomach. Sleep on your side with a pillow between your knees, or on your back. If you have a sore neck, go to a back specialty store and try out several neck pillows that reduce strain on your neck.

Notes

1. Kelsey, J.L., White, A.A. "Epidemiology and Impact on Low Back Pain." *Spine* 5 no. 2 (1980): 133–142.
2. National Council on Compensation Insurance.
3. Kelsey, J.L., White, A.A. "Epidemiology and Impact on Low Back Pain." *Spine* 5 no. 2 (1980): 133–142.
4. "The Effectiveness of Four Interventions for the Prevention of Low Back Pain." *Journal of the American Medical Association* 272 no. 16 (October 26, 1994).
5. ibid.
6. ibid.

PART 3

Doctors and Surgery

CHAPTER 7

When Should You Go to the Doctor... and Other Good Questions

If 80 percent of back pain goes away on its own over a month or so, when do you need the help of a doctor?

If you are covered under a managed care plan, you may already have access to a nurse for questions about back pain. Many large HMOs and PPOs (Preferred Provider Organizations) provide a nurse call line. These managed care organizations believe it makes good business sense to provide information to consumers so they can make intelligent decisions about their own care.

The Texas Back Institute continues to operate a nurse staffed phone line at 1-800-247-BACK. The nurses there can provide general information about your symptoms and offer some guidance to relieve your frustration or nervousness about your back or neck problem. They can also send you certain home remedies. If you have any serious symptoms, they will advise you to seek appropriate care in your local area.

Medical advice lines are now so commonplace that many hospital systems in large cities operate medical information phone lines. Some systems like "Ask-A-Nurse" are franchised medical advice systems that are operated in several cities around the country. For information in your area, check with your local hospital or HMO.

Typically, when you call a nurse medical advice line, the nurse will place your name and address in a computer so they can send you more information. Also, the nurse will ask you a series of questions to determine if you have any emergency symptoms. Remember, no one can diagnose your problem over the phone, not even a doctor, so don't expect that. You can receive helpful information about your specific symptoms and if you need to go to an Emergency Room, or if you can wait until the next day for an appointment with a physician.

Even if the phone line is not staffed by a nurse, the staff is trained to steer you to physician's offices that specialize in your problem. A good place to look is in the yellow pages for your city, under the heading for "hospitals" or "physicians and surgeons."

Using the phone for medical advice is not really new. The British medical journal *Lancet* notes that the first medical advice was provided over the phone in 1879. Not 1979, but 1879 — just three years after Alexander Graham Bell invented the telephone.

According to a healthcare analyst with Merrill Lynch, nurse-operated call centers are proliferating as a way to help control health care costs. It is estimated that the number of people who access call centers will grow from 35 million people currently to 100 million in the next four years. These call centers are helping people go to the correct place in the health care system. For example, 62 percent of those calling a nurse who would have gone to an Emergency Room were directed to a better alternative at a lower cost.

Can you diagnose yourself?

While an individual cannot reliably diagnose their own internal medicine or heart problems, a sore back is self-apparent. You may be interested to learn, however, that pain is a poor indicator of what is wrong with your back. A muscle strain, for example, can be more painful than a herniated disc.

When a back specialist examines you, she or he will be looking for other tell-tale symptoms that might imply a disc is affected. Pain that radiates from the back down into the leg, even into the bottom part of the leg, can imply a disc problem.

Another sign of a potential disc problem is called foot drop, where the patient is unable to raise the front of their foot. This muscle weakness may cause the person to drag the toe. Foot drop needs to be seen by a spine specialist immediately to prevent permanent nerve damage.

The worst symptom is cauda equina syndrome — loss of control of the bowel or bladder. If you notice this symptom, go to an emergency room immediately (the same day) to prevent permanent neurological damage and paralysis of bowel or bladder muscles. If doctors determine this symptom is caused by a disc problem, surgery will need to be done to prevent permanent damage to nerves.

Generally speaking, if you have any of the serious symptoms listed above, or have back pain that doesn't go away on its own after about three or four weeks, you may want to visit a spine physician just to rule out anything serious.

When should you go to the Emergency Room?

When it comes to back pain, the Emergency Room is often not the best place to go. For one thing, the doctor in an Emergency Room is usually a specialist in emergency medicine or occupational medicine. While you may get some immediate pain medication or muscle relaxants, you will probably be referred to a spine physician elsewhere for an appointment the next day. If you have back pain that is mostly in your lower back, without pain radiating into an arm or leg, you would be better off calling a spine specialist's office and telling them about the symptoms. Many times, especially if you are in extreme pain, the staff answering the phone at the spine doctor's office will squeeze you into the doctor's schedule.

A second reason to think twice about heading off to the Emergency Room for treatment of acute back pain is that your health insurance company may not pay for it because it is not a legitimate emergency in their view. Sure, you'll hand over your insurance card and the hospital staff will take the information down. But a month later, when your health insurance company sends you a bill for the entire Emergency Room visit, be prepared. You may just have a heart attack when you see the cost of using an Emergency Room!

Four important warning signs

1. **Loss of control of the bowel or bladder**

   Any time you have loss of control of the bowel or bladder, you should go to an Emergency Room or see a spine specialist the same day. This symptom represents "cauda equina syndrome" and there could be permanent neurological damage, or paralysis of your bowel and bladder muscles if you delay.

2. **Foot drop, weakness in the leg**

   Weakness that extends into your foot, especially if it is getting worse, may be a symptom is called "foot drop" and might call for a visit to the Emergency Room if you can't break into the spine specialist's schedule. Again, if you delay there could be permanent paralysis of the nerves involved and the weakness in your foot could be permanent. There are cases where people did not recognize that their leg symptoms were related to back injury and they delayed going to the doctor until too much time had passed. Once they were diagnosed, it was too late to repair the damage to the nerve root and they had to live with that symptom.

3. **Car accident or fall**

   Generally speaking, if you fall down stairs, are in an accident, slip, or have any other traumatic event that causes back or neck pain, you should go to an Emergency Room or see a spine specialist immediately. While most simple back pain doesn't need x-rays, when trauma is involved the doctor will need to take x-rays to make sure no vertebrae are fractured.

4. **Excruciating pain**

   If you are in excruciating pain, and it is in the evening or on the weekend, an Emergency Room may be your only alternative for relief. In this case, though, you might call the ER in advance. In some large hospitals the Emergency Room can resemble a war zone. While your back pain may be excruciating, your case may be low on the priority list compared to an incoming heart attack, laceration, or car wreck victim, and you may have to wait hours to see the emergency physician.

Doctors' biases

Unfortunately, as this book will explore in great depth, part of the problem with back pain is that there is a wide variety of back pain "experts" offering to help the back pain sufferer improve. Because each type of doctor brings along his or her treatment bias, it is important for the medical consumer to be well informed and to understand that every specialty that deals with back pain has a "dark side." Some of the things to keep in mind when you are involved with back care specialists are mentioned below.

Employers and insurers hate it that some chiropractors will perform weeks of chiropractic manipulation when it may not be doing any good. On the plus side, chiropractors can't legally prescribe drugs, so there is less risk of their over-medicating a back pain patient, which is the chief problem with general practice physicians who see back pain. Additionally, for some types of back pain, chiropractic manipulation can be very effective and the relief of pain can be instantaneous.

Spine surgeons — orthopedic or neurosurgeons — are trained to do surgery and, predictably, some of them are quick to recommend it. But they also may be the most knowledgeable about treating back pain because they see so much of it, and in some cases surgery may be the most prudent and economical solution of all.

A specialty that has gained a lot of attention in the last five years for treating back pain is "physical medicine and rehabilitation" (PMR). These PMR physicians, sometimes called "physiatrists," are experts in understanding how muscles work. Because 80 percent of back pain is muscle-related, these physicians are often best suited to treat back pain. A PMR physician, however, may perform unnecessary EMG (electromyography, see page 138) procedures or administer an excessive number of pain injections. Still, all of these activities are non-surgical and don't burn any bridges as thoroughly as surgery can do. All considered, among centers of excellence that specialize in spine care, PMR doctors are viewed as an ideal specialty for managing back and neck pain. If there is a surgical problem, the PMR physician will typically detect it quickly and refer it promptly to a competent spine surgeon.

What kind of back doctor should you see for an attack of acute pain?

Where is the best place to go for back care? That depends on the nature of your problem. Here are some resources to consider for an *acute* attack of back or neck pain. For chronic back or neck pain, where you have had the symptoms for more than three months, or if you have any emergency symptoms, go to the next category.

Primary care physicians There are a variety of specialists who see back pain. For simple back pain, a primary care physician — such as a family practice or internal medicine doctor — can do a competent physical evaluation and rule out serious problems.

If you work in a job involving heavy labor and have an injury that happened while at work, your supervisor may suggest that you go to an occupational medicine doctor. Because one-third of the accidents that happen on the job are back injuries, occupational medicine physicians can be very experienced in managing acute back or neck strain.

If there is any one primary care doctor most interested in your quick recovery, it is the occupational medicine doctor. Most "occ med" clinics depend on having excellent relations with nearby employers for future referrals. Because employers want their employees to return to work as soon as possible, occupational medicine physicians will strive to treat you quickly, get you into physical therapy — often the same day — and check on your progress.

Unfortunately, the same cannot be said all the time for primary care. Because there is a shortage of primary care doctors in most cities, you may find that it is harder to get an appointment to see a primary care doctor than to go right to a back specialist. Also, some primary care doctors may tend to emphasize a medication approach to treating back pain, rather than emphasizing physical therapy.

One complaint some large employers may have about primary care physicians seeing injured workers is that too many times the back pain sufferer is told by the generalist, "Take these pills and call me in two weeks if it still hurts." Consequently, some employers and workers compensation insurance carriers will steer injured workers directly to an occ med clinic, or directly to a physiatrist, orthopedic surgeon, or neurosurgeon who specializes in back and neck care. These providers are more likely to push the back strain patient to the therapist who will get the person moving again and back to activity as soon as possible.

Chiropractors As we have said, there is evidence that a chiropractor can provide good pain relief for acute back pain. Recent evidence shows that they may also be helpful in controlling symptoms for patients with chronic pain.[1, 2] If you have any red flag symptoms — like loss of control of the bowel, weakness of the leg, foot, or arm and hand — you should seek out an orthopedic surgeon or neurosurgeon. If you are seeing a chiropractor and these symptoms appear, you should expect him or her to obtain a consultation for you with a surgeon to ensure that there is no serious disorder that might require an operation.

The second benefit of chiropractic is that many times there is little waiting time before you can be seen for evaluation. Often, the chiropractor's schedule is flexible enough to work you in on the same or next day. Other benefits of chiropractic are that it doesn't emphasize a dependence on drugs to mask pain symptoms, and it is a non-surgical treatment alternative.

As with any procedure or treatment, you may want to check the coverage under your insurance plan and any restrictions or requirements you might need to meet. Treatment plans should be realistically focused on returning you to as pain-free and active a status as possible in a reasonable time frame. Beware of treatment plans that require you to keep coming back indefinitely for frequent manipulations.

Physiatrists Another good place to start might be the physical medicine and rehabilitation (PMR) specialists mentioned earlier in this chapter. Many managed care plans favor physiatrists because they are adept at treating back and neck pain with a variety of non-surgical options, including physical therapy and injections. PMR doctors also have a strong understanding of posture and gait and how this may affect back and neck strain.

Osteopathic physicians In theory, a Doctor of Osteopathy, or D.O., is a good blend between an M.D. and a chiropractor. Because D.O.s are able to prescribe drugs, like M.D.s, and have training in manipulation, like chiropractors, one would think they would be perfectly suited for treating back pain. Not all D.O.s do manipulation on their patients, however. One study found that, on average, only 18 percent of patients of D.O.s received manipulation.

Often, the geographic region in which you live dictates how osteopathic physicians are perceived in the medical community. In some locales D.O.s are perceived as a notch below M.D.s, but that is largely a regional bias. Some people believe osteopaths provide a healthy blend between traditional M.D.s and a more holistic approach to health care.

Orthopedic surgeons and neurosurgeons These two specialties are covered in detail in Chapter 10. Generally speaking, these two specialties are highly trained in treating all types of back pain — especially complex surgical cases. Because they are oriented toward surgery, some of the other physicians cited above may be better choices for simple, acute back pain.

Neurologists & rheumatologists Neurologists are experts in dealing with a variety of neurological disorders, including epilepsy, sleep disorders, brain disorders, headache, stroke, and chronic pain. Rheumatologists are experts in treating arthritis and other diseases affecting joints, muscles, bones, and tendons. Both specialties may become involved in your case if the other physicians listed above are unable to resolve your pain.

What kind of back doctor should you see for complex pain?

For complex back or neck symptoms that you have had for several months, or for complex emergency symptoms, it is better for you to search for a center that specializes in back pain. Typically, a spine center will include a multidisciplinary team of back care providers: doctors, physical therapists, exercise physiologists as well as access to diagnostics, injections, biofeedback, and chiropractic.

Within a spine center there may be several other types of specialists. Neurologists for example, focus on the nervous system, which includes the structure, functions, and abnormalities of the spine, brain, and nerve tissue. They can provide in-depth tests and evaluation of back pain to determine the root of the problem.

Most spine centers will be directed by either orthopedic surgeons or neurosurgeons. Both specialties are extremely experienced with treating the most complex cases imaginable.

The best spine centers focus exclusively on back and neck problems, that is, they don't treat knee, shoulder, or brain disorders. Look for a spine clinic where at least 75 percent of patients treated are there for back or neck pain.

Regina Herzlinger, a Harvard Business School professor, believes health care in the future will be transformed into clinics that specialize and have extensive experience in treating complicated problems. She envisions clinics that will cater to people suffering from particular ailments like asthma, diabetes, cancer, or spine problems, or in her words, "focused factories."

In Herzlinger's focused factories patients would find all the specialists they might need under one roof. Such is the case at several spine centers of excellence already in existence today. These centers combine skill sets like physical medicine and rehabilitation, neurosurgery, orthopedics, neurology, chiropractic, physical therapy, exercise physiology, psychologists, occupational therapists, athletic trainers, and hydrotherapists — all focused on back and neck problems.

If you go to this type of center, you will be assured of receiving the right type of care for your particular back problem.

How important is the doctor's personality?

It can be very important to find a doctor whom you can trust. If you end up with a physician who does not connect with you, or doesn't show genuine concern for your medical problem, you may not believe their recommendations and you may not stick with the therapy or treatment plan prescribed. Too many times patients give up on therapy before they give it a chance to work.

Secondly, it is important to find a doctor who takes the time to listen to you and hear about your back pain story — how you first got it and what it feels like. You are not a widget on an assembly line and shouldn't be treated as such. It is reasonable to expect the physician to spend at least 15 minutes with you in the exam room. For simple acute back pain, a physician shouldn't perform a lot of unnecessary x-rays and diagnostic tests because most back pain will get better on its own.

Once the physician performs the physical exam and begins to have an idea of what may be causing your problem, you should receive a thorough explanation of what may be causing your problem and what the doctor recommends as a next step. Keep in mind that at this point, after a preliminary examination, a doctor may still not know precisely what is causing your problem, and that is okay.

Don't misinterpret statements like, "First we will try a course of physical therapy to relieve pain, but if that doesn't work, we may then try . . ." Some people may think, "Do these doctors even know what they're doing?" The physician is not being indecisive, but rather is letting you know in advance that there are many alternatives to treating your back pain, and is involving you in the decision process.

Doctors are people, and they have their own personalities. Some older people like a doctor with an authoritative manner, who may appear decisive and confident and provide orders to be followed explicitly by the patient. Don't ask questions . . . just do it. You don't need to know why.

Other baby boomers find this style unappealing and prefer a physician who collaborates with the patient, taking time to make sure the patient understands the medical aspects of problem as well as the recommended treatment. The younger you are, the more likely you are to want to understand why physical therapy is supposed to work, before you commit to waking up at 6 A.M. for daily exercise sessions with the therapist.

To improve patient satisfaction, the Texas Back Institute appointment nurses often try to match new patients to a doctor based on the clinical problem as well as psycho-social factors. The patient can often give out cues as to the kind of doctor they would like. Sometimes a patient may note they are an avid runner or cyclist. There may be a physician who likes running or cycling who can then "connect" with the patient. By making a good match, nurses hope to increase the chances of a positive physician-patient interaction as well as increase the likelihood that the patient will then comply with the directives of the physician when it comes to attending therapy sessions and sticking with their customized home exercise regimen.

Government guidelines on treatment

Recognizing that spine care in the United States is a problem area, the U.S. Government commissioned the Agency for Health Care Policy and Research (AHCPR) to develop clinical guidelines. In the area of back pain, the AHCPR directed a multidisciplinary panel of physicians — surgeons, non-surgeons, chiropractors, and researchers — to review all the existing medical literature on various treatments for back pain. Their recommendations unsettled many surgeons who had become accustomed to seeing a patient on Monday, doing x-rays and diagnostics on the same visit, and scheduling the patient for surgical removal of a herniated disc later that same week.

The AHCPR guidelines recommended dramatic changes in the way physicians treat and diagnose back pain. Their premise is that most "simple" or uncomplicated back pain actually goes away on its own within six weeks. Further, physicians shouldn't even do x-rays within the first six weeks of care unless there are certain "red flag" neurological symptoms that imply something serious is involved. The AHCPR also recommended limited use of chiropractic manipulation in certain cases of simple back pain. Further, surgery should be the treatment of "last resort," and should be used only after a variety of non-surgical treatment alternatives are exhausted.

What kinds of things are done in the doctor exam?

A chiropractor may perform a slightly different physical exam and treatment than a medical doctor, although both will be trying to find clues that reveal the nature of your back problem. You may be asked to bend forward, backward, or sideways, walk on your heels or your toes.

An M.D. will also check for neurological signs by raising your leg and checking the strength in your foot, or the reflexes in your leg and foot, which may reveal pain symptoms or muscle weakness. One such test is the Babinski reflex. By stroking the bottom of your foot to see if your toes curl down the physician may determine that there is no damage to your spinal cord.

The doctor will ask questions about how and when your symptoms started, if they have changed, how you feel now, and what previous attacks of back pain you may have had. Next, the physician can perform various movements with your leg, raising it gently, moving your foot, all in ways that reveal significant information about your back and the spinal nerves. Through this exam the doctor will obtain 95 percent of the information needed to diagnose most spine problems.

It is crucial to answer the physician's questions accurately. Do not say there is pain when there is none, and be sure to tell the physician when a certain movement does create pain. Certain movements within this exam are designed to either produce pain or not produce pain, and your response gives the physician important diagnostic information about what may be causing your pain.

Diagnostic tests doctors do for back and neck pain

X-rays, scans and physician's exam The way physicians approach what is causing your back or neck pain is not unlike a detective finding out who murdered the butler during an evening dinner party. Like the detective, who is working with clues and a limited number of dinner guests who are suspects, the spine physician has a finite list of potential causes, and he or she will perform various tests to "rule out" various causes to arrive at the most likely one.

Sometimes, though, additional information is needed. Through x-rays, MRIs, and CT scans, a physician can look inside the body to help assess what is causing pain and what might be done to relieve it. All of these tests are painless. Combined with the physician's exam and your medical history, the physician can begin to get an idea of what may be going wrong. Your doctor may also order blood tests to rule out infection, inflammatory arthritis, and cancer. Physicians may also recommend urinalysis to rule out a kidney problem. Kidney stones, for example, can cause excruciating lower back pain.

In the past, it was commonplace for a physician to get x-rays for all back or neck pain patients. But now it is generally accepted practice to skip x-rays altogether unless you were in a fall or a car accident, or the doctor suspects a bone fracture from trauma.

But because x-rays only show bones, there is no way to see nerve root impingement or a bulging or herniated disc. The physician may suspect a disc problem, however, if the x-ray shows a smaller than normal space between the two vertebrae. This is called a "narrowing of the disc space," and might imply that the shock-absorbing disc is becoming squashed between two vertebrae.

CT scans (Computed Tomography) and MRI scans (Magnetic Resonance Imaging) can reveal soft tissue structures, such as ruptured discs, the spinal cord, narrowing of the spinal canal (stenosis), nerve roots, muscles, and bone. This is why x-rays are often skipped in favor of a more detailed CT or MRI scan. Your physician may have found during the physical exam that you have a problem which may need to be clarified through these specific tests.

During a CT or MRI scan, the patient lies still on a table that passes through the center of a large scanning device. A technician in another room operates the scanner with a computer to obtain the needed images. While x-rays and CT scans use radiation to view the inside of the body, MRI uses a magnetic field and a computer to produce its images. When MRI was first introduced, it was called nuclear magnetic resonance imaging, but the word nuclear had a bad connotation and so the technique was renamed.

An MRI machine is like a big magnet in the shape of a doughnut. A person lies on a table that slides inside the doughnut hole. This magnet can generate a magnetic force 20,000 times stronger that the earth's magnetic field, causing the molecules within the body to align themselves in specific directions. The MRI computer interprets this phenomena as images of tissues. This ability to provide the physician with images of soft tissues, including discs, is the main strength of MRI.

While MRI and CT scans are painless, some people may find it annoying or claustrophobic to lie perfectly still in an enclosed area for a half-hour or so. In some cases, a mild sedative can be prescribed.

Generally speaking, an MRI scan is more sensitive than a CT scan in evaluating nerve roots. An MRI can reveal if a disc has lost fluid or has ruptured. Tissues with high water content appear brighter, while aging or degenerated discs with less water appear darker. On the other hand, CT scans can be more helpful in evaluating subtle fractures.

Myelograms Myelography reveals additional diagnostic information about nerves and other spinal elements such as discs and bones, particularly when surgery is being considered. A physician injects dye into the spinal canal to enhance the radiological images.

Myelograms can show impingement from a herniated disc, bony overgrowth, spinal cord tumor, and spinal abscess. In a sense, it is like filling a hose with water and looking for constrictions.

During the procedure, the patient lies on a table that may be tilted to promote flow of the die into the desired area of the spine. The dye shows up as a white substance on x-rays, and herniated discs or bony overgrowths causing nerve impingement appear as obstructions where the dye is unable to surround the nerve root. MRIs have reduced the use of myelograms in recent years.

Patients should let their doctors know if they may be pregnant or if they are allergic to any medications or x-ray dyes, or if they are epileptic or diabetic. Afterward, patients usually spend four hours resting before going home. Side effects can include nausea, headaches, and infection at the injection site.

Discograms At the Texas Back Institute, physicians sometimes perform a pre-surgical test called a discogram. In this test a needle is used to inject a special dye into the herniated disc that is suspected of causing the person's back pain. An imaging device reveals if the dye travels outside of the disc space and near a nerve.

The purpose of this test is to actually recreate the back pain that may be caused by the suspicious disc. As a result the test can be painful, but it can also reveal if that specific disc is really the cause of the problem and if surgery is needed at all.

The worst possible scenario is to go through surgery, have a disc removed, only to wake to the horror that the back pain is still there and the disc that was removed was really not the problem at all.

EMGs EMGs (Electromyography) and Nerve Conduction Studies can be helpful in evaluating leg or arm weakness, numbness, pain, and cramping. If a patient has a herniated disc that is impinging upon a nerve root, a doctor can observe changes in specific leg muscles that signal radiating pain.

During an EMG, the physician inserts a fine needle electrode into various muscles. The needle may cause mild, temporary discomfort. By analyzing electrical activity on a screen and listening to sounds through a speaker, the physician can determine whether the muscle or the nerve to the muscle is working normally. During a Nerve Conduction Study, the physician tapes small metal electrodes on the skin and applies a brief electrical shock to the skin over a nerve. If the physician detects a slower than normal transmission, there may be a nerve disorder.

Bone Scan A bone scan can provide information about the possibility of tumor, infection, and arthritis or fracture in the bone and joints. In a bone scan an injection of radioactive material travels through the bloodstream and settles into bone, moving to areas that are metabolically active, indicating either bone destruction or bone formation. During the scan, the patient lies still on the a table as a camera passes back and forth across the body. If a fracture is new it appears as a "hot spot" on a bone scan, indicating ongoing metabolic activity in the region — the body's natural attempt to heal the break.

Notes

1. Triano, J., McGregor, M., Hondras, M., Brennan, P. "Manipulative Therapy Versus Education Programs in Chronic Low Back Pain." *Spine* 20 no. 8 (1995): 948–955.
2. Van Tulder, M.W., Koes, B.W., Bouter, L.M. "Conservative Treatment of Acute and Chronic Nonspecific Low Back Pain." *Spine* 22 no. 18 (1997): 2128–2156.

CHAPTER 8

The Pros and Cons of Back Surgery

This year, it is estimated that about 500,000 back and neck pain sufferers will be wheeled into surgical suites in hospitals across the United States for back and neck surgery. There, a surgeon will delicately cut out portions of a herniated disc to relieve painful pressure on nearby spinal nerves.

Experts agree that the procedure requires significant skill and practice, and is more complex than other types of joint surgery. That is because, unlike other joints and bones, the spine holds the spinal cord, the main electrical fusebox that controls the body.

When spine surgery goes well, the result is marvelous. A person can enter a surgical suite with excruciating pain and leave a couple of hours later relatively pain-free and ready to resume activity within days.

When spine surgery doesn't go well, however, it can be like someone dropped a metal wrench into that fusebox. In some cases the person may leave the surgical suite in worse condition than when they entered. Worse, in fact, because they now have a new problem, one that spine experts refer to as "failed back syndrome."

Like a massive short circuit, failed back syndrome can cause incessant pain that can puzzle the best spine specialists in the country.

Some spine experts theorize that by cutting around spinal nerves, the circulation to the area can be disrupted. Like a garden hose that is crimped, the slightly diminished circulation may be causing pain. Or the surgery may somehow cause certain areas to receive excessive circulation. The disc may continue to leak substances even after surgery, causing persistent pain and swelling.

Some doctors refuse to see a failed back patient, because they find them frustrating and difficult to help. Failed back patients often find themselves making pilgrimages from one doctor to another, ending up at large centers of excellence that specialize in such cases.

In the back business, a failed back patient is viewed as the most complex of all patients. They are likely to be referred from doctor to doctor until they end up with one who specializes in failed backs. This could be a physical medicine and rehabilitation physician, another surgeon, a pain specialist, or an anesthesiologist.

Because a physician may not be able to fix the short circuit, let alone determine where it is, failed back patients often have to rely on drugs to mask pain symptoms. The danger, in turn, of relying upon drugs to mask pain over a long period of time is that most drugs have potent side effects and can cause permanent and life-shortening damage to internal organs. In addition, such drugs can be addictive. As the body gets used to these drugs they become less effective and the dosage may need to be increased, which in turn raises the danger of side effects and complications. Hence, the failed back patient and failed back doctor face a dilemma: how can you relieve pain when you can't be sure anymore of what's causing it, and you can't use surgery or drugs to treat it?

For those employers and insurance companies who must pay the bill, the patience begins to wear thin after $30,000 has been spent on pain clinics and physician consults.

The patience of the failed back patient is most exhausted of all. These people are usually disabled by severe back pain and are out of work. This in turn places great strain on their family relationships. Some failed back patients are at the end of their rope, even considering suicide as the only permanent way of ending their pain. Masking the pain with heavy narcotics has also not been the answer. Failed back patients may have journeyed through aggressive rehabilitation programs, additional surgeries, injections, implantation of spinal cord stimulators and morphine pumps, and other last-ditch treatments aimed at relieving their pain.

Case in point: The Texas Back Institute in Dallas, Texas, is the nation's largest spine specialty clinic. It features fellowship-trained spine surgeons who specialize 100 percent in back and neck surgery. Those credentials understandably attract complex cases. Each year, the Texas Back Institute sees about 10,000 new back patients, of which about 2,000 — or one in five — are failed backs.

The Texas Back Institute is one of the few places that will treat failed back patients and wrestle with the complex challenge posed by the failed back case. Many cases that end up there are truly extreme.

What's so bad about surgery?

As the title implies, the intent of this book is to help a back or neck pain sufferer consider *all* the treatment alternatives before relying on surgery.

By reading this book, a back or neck pain sufferer will be empowered to discuss non-surgical resolutions for his or her problem intelligently with the doctor.

What's so bad about surgery? When done correctly and at the appropriate time, back surgery can be a godsend to the individual suffering from pain that sears into the leg or arm. For patients who are experiencing neurological symptoms like loss of control of the bowel or bladder, surgery is necessary to prevent permanent paralysis. Patients with foot drop often must have back surgery performed quickly to prevent permanent nerve damage. Fortunately, these cases of emergency back surgery are not too common.

Unlike heart patients, who often stand to get worse or develop complications the longer heart surgery is delayed, most back patients have time on their side. With the exception of those patients with the neurological complications mentioned above, many herniated discs will go "asymptomatic" — that is, their pain symptoms will disappear — if given enough time.

That may be small comfort to someone who is suffering excruciating back pain because of a herniated disc. The prospect of waiting a weekend, let alone six weeks, may be too much. Depending upon the extent of herniation, the pain can be unbearable if not treated.

Fortunately, there are non-surgical treatment alternatives that can help the patient get through some of the pain symptoms and give Mother Nature a chance to do her magic.

But why wait anyway? Why not rush into surgery if it will provide instantaneous relief?

The dangers of surgery are considerable. First, there are the risks of any surgical procedure, however small, such as the chance of complications during anesthesia or surgery. Medicare reports that for every 1,000 patients over 65 years of age undergoing back fusion surgery, 14 will die within 30 days. Many reputable spine specialists discourage patients above 70 from having elective spine surgery because the risks may outweigh the potential benefits.

How many spine surgeries end up as "train wreck" failed backs? While heart surgery has mortality statistics, and cancer treatment has benchmark statistics for five-year survival rates, in the spine field there are few hard statistics. Consequently, at this time there really isn't good data to quantify the odds of your spine surgery turning out poorly.

The possibility of ending up a failed back patient is a scary proposition. Even a simple disc surgery patient, in good health, could wheel through the doors of the surgical suite and then wheel out the same doors two hours later, only to end up in that horrible purgatory of failed back syndrome.

While it is fair to say that most patients emerge from simple spine surgery greatly improved, the odds of a successful surgery are linked to four variables:

1. accurate diagnosis of the problem
2. the severity of the problem
3. the patient's physical condition and health going into surgery
4. the surgeon performing the surgery

Variable number 4 relates to the premise that the more experienced the spine surgeon, the more likely there will be a positive outcome.

Generally speaking, if you have a herniated disc that has an obvious protrusion or free floating fragment that is clearly impinging on a nearby nerve, chances are very good that your surgery will have a good outcome.

If your case is less clear cut and the physician isn't sure about the cause of the pain, or if the pain is mostly in your back area, the surgery may not achieve the desired pain-relieving result. In some cases, you might end up worse.

For those back or neck pain sufferers who have no option — who could suffer permanent paralysis or nerve complications — Chapter 10 goes into detail about how to improve your odds if you need spine surgery.

Excessive surgeries

Surgeons are trained to cut. Consequently, many surgeons simply believe that the best way to treat back pain from a herniated disc is to cut out the herniation.

In reality, however, studies show that at least half of those people who have back pain from herniated discs will get better without surgery — with time and non-surgical treatment. Outcome studies, for example, show that herniated disc patients treated with surgery really aren't any better off five and 10 years later than those treated non-surgically.

In the medical practice business, a doctor's inventory is his or her time. If time is not used productively, it is lost and cannot be recovered. Some surgeons view the days they spend seeing patients in their office as time spent culling patients to fill their surgical schedule. If they have six surgical slots a week to fill for a full schedule, their intent may be to fill those slots to make for a productive week. If you are seen during a week where the schedule is light, the likelihood of getting on a surgery schedule might go up dramatically.

This highlights a benefit to going to a spine center of excellence for a complex back problem. The best spine physicians usually have a two week waiting period before they can see a new patient, although emergencies are seen on the same day. Expert spine surgeons may have a two or three month waiting period before a new case can get on their surgery schedule. This wait, while painful, works to your benefit. The longer your wait on the surgery schedule, the more chance your back pain will improve before your surgery day arrives.

Despite the above scenario, the incidence of unnecessary back surgery in the United States should not all be blamed on over-zealous back surgeons. We are a consumer-oriented culture, and health care is also a consumer service. Sometimes unnecessary back surgeries are driven by patient demand for relief of extreme pain, where the surgeon feels pressured or moved by the impassioned requests of the back pain sufferer.

In one such case, the wife of a senior executive of a corporation arrived at the Texas Back Institute with excruciating back pain. The surgeon decided that surgery needed to be delayed. The wife called her husband, who in turn had the company's health benefits manager pressure the Texas Back Institute to "expedite" surgery for this VIP. The surgeon explained that the woman's case was not ready for surgery and she was being managed appropriately with injection therapy to relieve pain. He was proven right. Over three days of non-surgical care the woman's symptoms improved and eventually she recovered from the episode without the need for surgery.

An incident like this underscores why a spine center needs to have objective criteria for performing back surgery. Most spine centers have some type of review system to double-check or approve cases before they get on a surgery schedule. The Texas Back Institute has such a pre-surgical review system, where upcoming surgeries are screened by peer surgeons — and non-surgeons — before they are approved for surgery. If someone has not had six weeks of non-surgical care beforehand, they are usually removed from the surgery schedule.

Back surgery in other cultures

Our perspective in the United States is often slanted. As a culture, we often look for a quick fix: a pill or a surgery to immediately make pain symptoms go away. For example, the rate of people undergoing back surgery in other countries differs dramatically from that the United States. One researcher notes that European countries like Great Britain, Sweden, and Finland do half as much spine surgery as in the United States.[1] Even within the United States there is great disparity in surgical rates. 60 percent more spine surgery is performed in the Southern states than in the Western states.[2] Some theorize that is because doctors train in regional centers and then settle nearby, practicing with the same bias as the medical school and residency program that trained them. Others theorize that managed care, which has its roots in California, has trimmed the surgical rate in that area.

Within the United States, some experts estimate that almost half of back and neck surgeries are unnecessary. Researchers at the Rand Corporation, for example, estimate that 40 percent of laminectomies are unnecessary. Another research firm, MediQual, reported in 1991 that about 50 percent of the laminectomies they studied didn't have objective clinical findings documented in the hospital medical record to validate the need for back surgery.

Physician, first do no harm Some studies on back pain reveal that some patients are worse after treatment than before — an indicator of wide treatment variation and questionable quality in the spine care field.[3] A lot of surgeons will recommend surgery — in some cases extensive surgery involving bone grafts and fusion of the vertebrae — on the basis of their personal bias toward surgical treatment.

Changing these attitudes can be difficult. While current back research is filled with literature that shows repeat back surgery rarely produces improvement, many patients have a series of back surgeries. As noted earlier, one patient arrived at the Texas Back Institute with 24 previous back surgeries performed elsewhere!

There are many ways to improve the situation. Having physicians use non-surgical clinical protocols to reduce treatment variation, and then collecting clinical outcome data, would enable researchers to compare centers. By finding the best treatments, researchers could then make broad recommendations to physicians as to the best treatments for back pain.

Risk from the surgeon It's okay to develop a trusting relationship with your doctor. Just remember that if your doctor is a surgeon by training, he or she will have a natural bias toward using surgery as a way of resolving your back or neck pain. Surgeons, generally speaking, are action oriented, often confident in their abilities, and eager to help the patient become pain-free.

Also remember that the surgeon may be using your pain complaints as a guide to how bad the herniated disc may be. No doctor wants to see their patient in unbearable pain. Consequently, for your own benefit, you would be well served to not exaggerate your pain symptoms. To get a clearer understanding of your pain, doctors may ask you to rate the pain on a zero to ten scale, with zero being no pain at all and ten being unbearable, "put-me-out-of-my-misery" pain.

One of the risks involved in back surgery is related to how many times the surgeon has performed the specific procedure. Many doctors argue vocally against using this as a criterion, saying that just because a doctor only does 25 spine surgeries a year doesn't make him or her a bad surgeon. Perhaps.

Medicare's mortality statistics have shown that hospitals that performed a small number of heart surgeries had higher than normal deaths. A growing number of employers and managed care companies also believe the old adage that "practice makes perfect" does indeed apply, and that the number of back surgeries performed by a surgeon can help determine her or his proficiency, provided the surgeries were appropriate and the surgeon had a history of good outcomes.

Some large employers have created specialty networks that include the super-specialists in categories like spine or hip surgery. In developing these networks, more and more employers use what is called "volume credentialing" to eliminate the surgeons who perform a small number of surgeries. Why? Because more data is emerging that, just like any other skill, the more you do something the better you get at it.

Under volume credentialing, a physician must do a minimum "volume" of surgeries to be credentialed as an expert. In the spine field, an orthopedic surgeon or neurosurgeon whose practice is 100 percent spine-related may do about 150–200 or more spine surgeries a year. Some large purchasers of healthcare require that a surgeon perform at least 100 spine surgeries a year to be considered expert.

Everybody knows that practice makes perfect. But have you considered asking your surgeon how many back or neck surgeries she or he does a year? Ask.

It is hard to be good without practice. James G. Jollis, a cardiologist at Duke University Medical Center, revealed a study in 1997 that showed the more angioplasties performed by a doctor, the lower the complication rate. In angioplasty, a tiny balloon is inserted into a blocked heart artery and inflated to clear the obstruction. The study showed that doctors who perform a lower number of angioplasties have a higher incidence of complications. Dr. Jollis estimated that at least 1,200 Medicare patients a year have adverse outcomes as a result of using physicians with insufficient experience.

The American Heart Association and the American College of Cardiology both recommend that cardiologists who do angioplasties should perform at least 75 a year or stop doing them.

Who must have spine surgery — quickly Generally speaking, if you have loss of control of the bowel or bladder and may have the disorder called "cauda equina syndrome," you require surgery quickly.

If you have weakness in a leg or foot that is getting worse, there may be a need for surgery relatively quickly as well. Nerve root compression often will cause weakness or numbness in an arm or leg. When that weakness or numbness worsens, it is called "progressive nerve root compression" or "progressive motor weakness." As long as your spine physician sees your symptoms improving rather than getting worse, non-surgical treatment can be continued for up to 12 weeks, and you may be able to postpone surgery with the hope that your symptoms may go away completely.

Delaying surgery for cauda equina syndrome or progressive motor weakness could result in permanent nerve damage that could cause you to have permanent loss of bowel or bladder control, or permanent weakness in a leg or arm. Thus the importance of acting quickly on these symptoms.

Spine tumors, or other rare abnormalities in the spine, may also need immediate surgery. While spine tumors are very rare, the seriousness of these tumors underscores why it is a good idea to visit a back doctor for any back or neck pain symptom that does not go away on its own after a couple of weeks of home remedies. A simple physical exam by the doctor can alleviate most concerns and get you on your way with a long-term home exercise program. It's hard to put a price on peace of mind like that.

Together, all of the above emergency back surgeries account for less than 5 percent of back surgeries.

Can your spine surgery wait? In probably 95 percent of cases, back surgery is an elective procedure, meaning it could be delayed without complications. In fact, as explained, delaying the surgery gives time for the symptoms to disappear, which can indeed happen. This explains why some managed care companies are developing guidelines that mandate a six-week waiting period before back surgery, during which non-surgical options are explored and given a chance to work.

Even without weakness in a leg or arm, delaying surgery can mean living with severe pain for several weeks. Some people simply can't endure this pain.

Others, like professional athletes who have time working against them in their finite career spans, often feel pressure to surgically repair the problem and accelerate their recovery. They cannot wait for a non-surgical cure to work because they may lose their contract and their spot on a professional sports team. An injury that takes a year to heal may, for all practical purposes, be career-ending for them.

Keep in mind the following, however. These athletes are in fantastic shape going into surgery, are geared to withstand the painful workouts associated with aggressive rehabilitation after surgery, are going to the nation's best (and most-sought-after and expensive) surgical specialists, and have to be back in top shape in only a couple of months to earn a living at their career. Can you say the same for yourself?

Most people do not need to be back by January to quarterback their team in the Super Bowl. Most people are going back to a forklift seat, a loading dock, or a computer screen. Also, in many cases, a person will end up with a surgeon who does less than 30 spine surgeries a year, instead of 200. Lastly, how many of us are really in great physical shape heading into the operating room, let alone have the drive to endure daily rehab workouts afterward?

Do you need back surgery?

Everyone with back pain eventually wants to know if they have a problem that may require back surgery. If you don't have any of the emergency symptoms described above, then you don't need surgery now. Some people presume that surgery is always an option, a last-ditch way to relieve back or neck pain. That is not necessarily the case. In 80 percent of back or neck pain cases, such as muscle-related pain, surgery is never an appropriate alternative.

Here are some guidelines to determine if you have a type of problem that may potentially require surgery down the road.

Surgery may be appropriate when . . .

1. You have had an MRI, CT scan, or myelogram and your doctor has concluded that you indeed have a herniated disc *and* it is also impinging on a nearby nerve *and* that specific nerve corresponds with the pain symptoms you are experiencing. (The key word here is "and." A lot of people have herniated discs and have no back pain at all. There are also cases where a surgeon has removed a herniated disc at one level in the spine, only to have the patient wake up after surgery and find the pain is still there because that specific disc was not the pain generator. Also, a herniation does *not* mean a bulge. Surgery is not needed for bulging discs. Herniation means the disc wall has broken and the disc is protruding outward — pushing on a nerve.)

2. You have pain that radiates down your leg or arm past your knee or elbow.

3. You have weakness or tingling in your foot.

4. With all the above, when you lie down and try to raise your leg, there is increased pain in your *leg* rather than in your lower back. That's right. If the pain gets worse in your back when doing a straight leg raise, that's probably *not* an indicator for surgery. Ironically, if you have a surgical problem, a straight leg raise will cause pain in a leg, not the back.

Surgery may *not* be appropriate when . . .

1. Your back or neck pain is mostly in your back and neck, and it doesn't radiate into a leg or arm.

2. You haven't tried physical therapy, or another form of conservative care, for six weeks.

If you don't have any red flag danger symptoms that require emergency surgery, ask yourself if you can tolerate the pain a little longer. Those extra days may give Mother Nature that time she needs to work her magic and to make your pain lessen and eventually go away. It's not unusual that, over time, many cases of herniated disc will eventually stop hurting. This doesn't mean the problem has gone away permanently, but if you are careful in the future, you can manage and live through any recurrences. Similarly, even if you were to have back surgery, it is no guarantee that you won't have a similar problem develop afterward.

In summary, if you are a back surgery candidate, determine if it is elective or emergency surgery. If it is elective, then elect to take your time with your decision.

Notes

1. Frymoyer, J.W., ed. "The Epidemiology of Spinal Disorders." *The Adult Spine: Principles and Practice* (New York: Raven Press, 1991).
2. Taylor, V.M., Deyo, R.A., Cherkin, D.C., Kreuter, W. "Low Back Pain Hospitalization: Recent United States Trends and Regional Variations." *Spine* 19 no. 11 (1994): 1207–1213.
3. Grubb, S.A., Lipscomb, Gilford, W.B. "The Relative Value of Lumbar Roentgenograms, Metrizamide, Myelography and Discography in Patients with Chronic Low-Back Syndrome." *Spine* 12 (1987): 282–286.

CHAPTER 9

What Actually Happens in Back Surgery

Types of back surgery

Sometimes surgery is necessary to prevent paralysis. Sometimes it offers quick and dramatic relief from severe pain. If you are one of the estimated 500,000 people having back surgery this year, here is some information on common procedures your back surgeon might use to correct problems in the spine.

Discectomy During a traditional discectomy, a spine surgeon removes a portion of a herniated disc — typically, the portion that is pressing on a nearby nerve — through a two- to three-inch incision while the patient is under general anesthesia. The undamaged portion of the disc is usually left in place to continue to act as a shock absorber.

Microdiscectomy As you learn about back surgery, you may hear the term microdiscectomy. The term relates to the use of a microscope during back surgery. In some patients, the disc herniation may be in an area that allows the surgeon to make a small incision and pluck out the herniated part of the disc. Unfortunately, not all herniated discs can be operated on this way. Often, the vertebrae shield the disc from the view of the surgeon. Many times, the herniation will be in an area that is not easy for the surgeon to reach unless there is an open incision and part of the lamina is removed. Consequently, many surgeons prefer a traditional open incision. Their philosophy is to do the surgery correctly the first time to prevent the need for a second operation.

Percutaneous discectomy Similar to microdiscectomy, percutaneous discectomy promised to completely change the field of back surgery when it was introduced in the late 1980s. In fact, the Texas Back Institute was one of 19 centers in the United States first approved to perform the procedure when it was introduced.

In this procedure, the surgeon makes a small half-inch incision in the lower back that can later be covered with a Band-Aid. Using a surgical probe the width of a ball point pen, the surgeon maneuvers the end of the probe near the herniated disc. In the tip of the probe are tiny scissors that can cut and remove the herniated disc tissue. Early probes had a fiber-optic camera that enabled the surgeon to guide the probe into position. Once in position, the camera lens was replaced with the cutting blades. The Texas Back Institute and other centers found, however, that like microdiscectomy, percutaneous discectomy only works well for certain disc herniations that are located in an area that the surgeon can reach with the probe.

The Texas Back Institute found that percutaneous discectomy did not have the success rate of traditional back surgery. While there are centers that advertise "Band-Aid" back surgery, many expert spine surgeons feel that the success rate of the procedure poses the risk that a surgeon may have to perform a second surgery to get the job done right. Our opinion is that, in general, the risk of a second procedure, along with the second anesthesia, doesn't warrant taking the chance with the technique.

A couple more caveats about percutaneous discectomy: first, not all patients qualify for the procedure. Appropriate patients may include those who have not had previous back surgery and whose leg pain is worse than their back pain. Second, any patient considering percutaneous discectomy should ensure their surgeon has had adequate training in the procedure and adheres to its strict patient selection criteria.

Laser discectomy This is a procedure similar to percutaneous discectomy, first tested in 1991. Instead of a mechanical probe, the surgeon uses laser energy to vaporize disc material. Both percutaneous and laser discectomies are typically performed with the patient under local anesthesia. While percutaneous discectomy can be beneficial in appropriate patients, in the authors' opinion, laser discectomy is of extremely limited value. As with any type of percutaneous procedure, the herniation has to be in a position that the probe can reach, which is not possible if the herniated area is protected by part of the bony vertebrae.

Laminectomy In a laminectomy, a spine surgeon makes a one- to two-inch incision in the lower back. The surgeon then chips away the lamina of one or more vertebrae to gain access to the disc area. Any fragments that may have broken away from the disc, as well as the area of disc that is herniated and pressuring a nerve root, is then removed. Since, if the entire disc were removed, you would lose the shock absorbing function of the disc between the vertebrae, the surgeon will typically remove that part of the disc that has ruptured outward along with another 10 or 20 percent to prevent future problems arising.

Fusion Sometimes surgeons, generally orthopedic surgeons, will recommend a fusion surgery. It may be that your doctor suspects that there is some instability or motion in your spinal vertebrae that is causing pain. Or it may be that you have a herniated disc that is pressuring a nearby nerve root. When the disc is removed, then the vertebral segment may become unstable. The solution to that instability may be to make a small bone graft, sometimes from your own pelvis or sometimes from sterile bone that comes from a bone donor (typically a cadaver).

Whether you need a fusion or not depends on the extent of the disc damage and whether your surgeon feels she or he can remove the troublesome portion of the disc but still retain stability in the vertebrae without any fusion or instrumentation.

Should you care? In our opinion, any time you hear the word "fusion" you should investigate more closely and probably get a second opinion, just as you should with any surgical recommendation.

There are many different types of fusion – some from the front, others from the back, some with instruments, and others without. It is important that you thoroughly understand the procedure, why it is being proposed, and the potential complications.

Spine surgeries involving a fusion are generally quite complicated. A 1994 study of lumbar fusion patients in Washington State revealed that 89 of 388 lumbar fusion patients — 23% — had another lumbar spine operation within two years, of which 40% involved removal of prior instrumentation such as plates, rods, screws, etc. Of the total number of fusion patients studied, 68 percent felt that their back or leg pain was worse after surgery, and 56 percent said that their overall quality of life was no better or worse.

About 62 percent of the patients said they would go through the surgery again, but those were mostly the ones who eventually returned to work. For example, four-and-a-half years after their surgery, only 41 percent of patients were working. Researchers also theorized that, while the intent of using instrumentation is to reduce the need for subsequent surgery, in reality the presence of instrumentation increased the odds of needing a second surgery.[1]

It is important to note that this study involved patients who were injured on the job and were receiving workers compensation payments for being off work. Those who deal with work-related back injuries often note that when a person is receiving compensation for back disability there can be a motive for secondary gain.

Managed care organizations who review spine surgeries are concerned when they see a doctor recommending fusion surgery. The above study also notes that there is a ninefold regional variation in rates of lumbar fusion surgery in the United States.

This study and many others are raising doubts about the use of fusion in back surgery. As a result, in Washington state the number of such surgeries decreased from 1.6 fusions per 1,000 population in 1987 to 1.2 fusions per 1,000 population five years later.[2]

This does not mean that you should automatically say no to a fusion, just that you should always get a second opinion before going forward.

Foramenotomy The foramina are the small openings in the bony vertebrae through which the spinal nerves exit the spinal cord on their way to other parts of the body. Over time, as the spine becomes more susceptible to degenerative changes, bony overgrowths, and conditions like narrowing of the spinal canal, the space for the nerve roots can become restricted. During a foramenotomy, the surgeon carefully shaves bone around the foramina to free up space for the nerves and to decrease irritation and inflammation.

Chymopapain You don't hear much about chymopapain anymore. About 10 years ago, some spine doctors injected chymopapain, an enzyme found in the papaya plant, into the disc space to dissolve a herniated disc. The procedure fell out of favor, however, when several patients had serious complications. Some experts theorize that the procedure itself wasn't the problem, rather the doctors performing it. In any event, few doctors recommend or use the procedure currently.

Neuroablation and Rhizotomy Techniques Neuroablation is an umbrella term relating to destruction of a nerve that may be transmitting a pain signal. In rhizotomy, for example, a spine surgeon may try to relieve facet joint pain by cutting the nerves of the vertebral facet joint, thereby interrupting the facet joint's ability to transmit pain. A rhizotomy is usually performed on an outpatient basis, using local anesthesia and intravenous sedation.

Nerves can also be destroyed with extreme heat and cold, which is called thermal neuroablation. An anesthesiologist, for example, may use a needle probe to locate the offending nerve and then apply extreme cold or extreme heat through the end of the probe to either freeze the nerve or burn it. Either way, the physician is attempting to interrupt the pain signal from the nerve to the brain. In general, rhizotomy tends to be more permanent, while the effects of freezing or burning may last six months or so.

Rhizotomy and neuroablation techniques are something in-between conservative care and back surgery. They are intended to provide a bridge back to activity and exercise. Because the results are sometimes erratic and involve complications, these treatments should be used selectively.

Scoliosis surgery Scoliosis, a condition that causes the spine to develop a sideways curve, and kyphosis, where the upper back curves forward, can sometimes be severe enough to require surgical correction.

As mentioned previously, most young patients with scoliosis can be treated with bracing to arrest or slow down the progression of their spinal curves. Curvature that reaches about 40 degrees before a child reaches skeletal maturity can be expected to progress and cause possible health problems in adults, including dangerous crowding of the heart and lungs in the most serious cases.

Spinal curvatures can be treated in children or adults by surgeons who specialize in spine deformity surgery, using metal hook-and-rod instrumentation systems such as Cotrel-Dubousset or TSRH, which offer better correction of scoliosis curves than older techniques such as Harrington Rods. Once the spine is straightened, the surgeon grafts bone in place so that the corrected curve will fuse into the straightened position. Patients usually wear plastic braces as the fusion heals.

Spinal tumor surgery Fortunately, tumors in the spine are rare. When detected, they can be treated with radiation, surgery, or both. Surgical treatment might include removal of the tumor and fusion to stabilize the area.

Surgery from the front or back A significant consideration in elective surgery is which approach the surgeon will use to reach the herniated disc or perform the fusion. The surgeon may use an anterior approach, that is, make an incision in the abdomen or at the front of the neck. In the posterior approach, the physician makes an incision in the lower back, or at the back of the neck. When an anterior (frontal) approach to lower back surgery is used, there may be a general surgeon involved who will make the incision in the abdomen and move aside all the internal organs and arteries so the spine surgeon can see the spine.

The latest advances in spine surgery

In the 1990s there have been a tremendous number of exciting advances that have improved clinical outcomes from back surgery. Typically, the most advanced types of spine surgery are only available at spine specialty centers because of the degree of training needed to perform the surgery.

Typically, the arthroscope is a long, hollow tube that contains a fiber-optic camera lens and a light source. The surgeon sees the operative site through one small incision and operates via two other small incisions.Just as arthroscopic surgery has revolutionized shoulder and knee treatment, new approaches are being explored in spine surgery. Thanks to the arthroscope orthopedic surgeons can repair damaged tissue through tiny incisions rather than making long, open incisions that require a longer recovery time after surgery.

Dr. John Regan at the Texas Back Institute was one of the first surgeons in the nation to pioneer a new surgical technique called Video-Assisted Thoracotomy (VAT).

Traditionally, the most complicated spine surgery involves the thoracic spine, the middle area of the spine behind the heart. Those people who needed anterior surgery on their thoracic spine needed a large incision and a team of surgeons to navigate past key arteries to reach the spine. The incision, along with the spreading of the rib cage, stretching of nerve tissue, and cutting of muscle required to reach the thoracic spine usually meant a week or more in the hospital and a long, three month recovery period.

Using the new Video-Assisted Thoracotomy procedure, instead of a large incision and spreading the rib cage, the surgeon can delicately maneuver the surgical probe through a few small incisions and perform the repair work with the aid of a video monitor. During VAT, television monitors are placed at the head of the table, on either side of the patient. Through the incision the surgeon inserts a scope with a lens and fiber-optic cable to light the area and transmit video to the television monitors. Two additional small incisions are made above and below the scope site to serve as working portals through which the surgeon inserts surgical instruments. Patients usually leave the hospital about two days after VAT surgery and return to activity in four to six weeks.

For the patient, Video-Assisted Thoracotomy is thought to represent far less risk from surgery, a shorter time in the hospital, and a shorter recovery period.

New technology and instrumentation

The artificial disc Just as heart surgeons have dreamed of inventing an artificial heart, spine surgeons have tried to develop an artificial disc that can be used to replace a damaged one. These new artificial discs have already been implanted successfully in spine patients in Europe, and are awaiting FDA approval for use in the United States. For those people with degenerative disc disease, where several discs in their spine are degenerating, a workable artificial disc would be a godsend.

Fixation cages, screws, plates, and rods When a spine becomes unstable because of a fracture or badly damaged disc, spine surgeons may have to fuse bone grafts or apply plates and screws to secure the vertebrae and prevent movement after surgery. New fixation cages are now available that may help to make instrumentation surgery more successful.

Scoliosis surgery, to straighten a curved spine, is constantly going through evolution, with new systems continually being introduced for better curve correction with less risk. The scoliotic spine actually resembles a bent corkscrew, something that is not only bent over but also twisted. Older Harrington Rod systems, which were the state-of-the-art technology during the 1970s, merely straightened the spine without untwisting it. These have now been mostly replaced by rod systems that attach hooks to individual vertebrae and enable the surgeon to "de-rotate" the curved spine and achieve a far better correction with less complications.

Pedicle screws and other "experimental" surgeries If your head is beginning to swim, that is understandable. But there is more. If you are undergoing surgery, you will have to sign an informed consent form at or before the time of surgery. Most reputable spine centers will provide you with the form as well as a thorough educational video days before the surgery, so you don't feel pressured.

If your surgery is a fusion, and your surgeon intends to use pedicle screws to assist in the fusion, your informed consent form might state that your surgeon is using hardware that is not approved by the FDA. The FDA (Food and Drug Administration) is a U.S. agency that regulates the use of new drugs and surgical equipment in the United States.

Briefly, pedicle screws are used to hold bone fusions in place and increase the likelihood that your fusion surgery is successful. They are also a source of many lawsuits in the United States. Detractors criticize them because some people have had complications from surgery involving pedicle screws. Advocates argue that if you don't use them, chances are increased that the fusion surgery will be a failure.

Critics of the FDA are also quick to point out that the FDA may often stand in the way of approving beneficial drugs and surgical equipment that could save lives and improve surgical outcomes. Getting FDA approval for a new drug or surgical device may take years in the United States. That is why European countries are often the first to implement new technology. In defense of the FDA, it is their job to try and reduce the chance of releasing a potentially harmful drug or device for use on American consumers.

Spine surgeons find themselves in a difficult position on this issue. If they don't use a pedicle screw and the surgery is a failure they could be questioned as to why they didn't use pedicle screws — technology that is largely regarded in the industry as a standard treatment. If they do use pedicle screws and there is a complication, they have a different set of circumstances to address.

Multiple spine surgeries

Sometimes a person can have one spine surgery, and still not be better. In the spine industry this is technically labeled a failed back. A failed back patient represents a major challenge for a spine center.

Needing a second surgery may not necessarily mean that the first surgery was a failure, however, but that additional surgery is needed to repair a new problem at a different level in the spine.

There is some research in the spine field that covers multiple operations and their success rate. In one study of failed back surgery patients who had a second surgery, about one-third were better afterward. Depending upon your perspective, a salvage rate of one-third may be good news. On the other hand, the researchers also noted that of the other two-thirds studied, some patients got worse, although they couldn't be sure worsening of their condition wouldn't have happened even if they hadn't had a second surgery. The researchers did find that younger patients had a better chance of improvement with a second operation than the older patients in the study.[3]

Recovery after spine surgery

For simple, uncomplicated back or neck surgery, you may spend one or two nights in the hospital. In some cases, you may be able to go home the same day. Even if you stay in the hospital, your doctor may encourage a speedy recovery. The Texas Back Institute, for example, has their own physical therapists working in the hospital. The morning after back surgery, a therapist will get the patient up out of the bed and moving up and down the hall. While great care is taken to protect the surgical incision, the therapists will encourage the patient to start gentle movements so their muscles don't atrophy and become stiff. After you are home, your doctor will likely have you participate in a post-surgical rehabilitation program. You will attend therapy sessions for two to four weeks as you regain strength, flexibility, mobility, and most of all, confidence in your abilities.

Surgery involving fusion, or instrumentation to stabilize vertebrae or correct spinal deformity will often require several days in the hospital and a longer recovery period. Unlike simple back surgery patients, those patients with fusions will have very limited activity because the focus will be on allowing the bone graft to fuse properly.

Notes

1. Johnson, S.M., Jurtz, M.E., Kurtz, J.C. "Variables Influencing the Use of Osteopathic Manipulative Treatment in Family Practice." *Journal of the American Osteopathic Association* (1997): 80–87.
2. "Outcome of Lumbar Fusion in Washington State Workers' Compensation." *Spine* 19 no. 17: 1897–1904.
3. "Failed Back Surgery Syndrome: 5 year follow up in 102 Patients Undergoing Repeated Operation." *Neurosurgery* 28 no. 5 (1991).

CHAPTER 10

Finding the Best Surgeon

As we have said repeatedly in this book, a back or neck pain sufferer should not rush into surgery. There are times, however, when surgery is unavoidable because of dangerous symptoms. Also, if you have exhausted most of the nonsurgical alternatives for treating your back and neck pain, your physician may advise that it's time to consider surgery. Consider this a crucial decision point.

Up to now, your physicians may have examined you and prescribed simple remedies or administered pain-relieving injections. Up to now, the risk of something going wrong because of your care was relatively low. With surgery, however, the stakes change. The treatment is more invasive and the results are permanent. Don't base your decision on how confident the surgeon is about performing the particular surgery you need. Surgeons by nature must be confident to be good at their trade. Remember, though, the surgeon doesn't have to live with the result — you do.

With this in mind, you should now go about the process of locating the best possible surgeon for your back or neck surgery, because your selection will have a great deal to do with your outcome. Managed care organizations who track complication rates and outcomes can testify that not all surgeons are created equal.

If your surgeon needed back surgery for something out of his or her area of expertise, you can be assured he or she would research the best surgeon in the field and go there. They would not resign themselves to the most conveniently located doctor. If the best possible care isn't located in your area, be ready to travel.

Most major cities will have many competent back surgeons. The same may not be true for smaller cities of 100,000 people or less. Only five orthopedic surgeons and one or two neurosurgeons would be needed for a city this size. Will one of these seven doctors be the best choice for you? If your spine surgery is relatively simple, perhaps one of these surgeons will be fine. If your spine surgery is somewhat complex, needing instrumentation or bone fusions to stabilize the spine, the best surgeon for you may be three hours away in a larger metropolitan area.

Typically, the best and brightest surgeons live in attractive and desirable areas. For example, North Dallas is a very desirable place to live. As a result, there are 15 orthopedic surgeons per 100,000 people — three times the number needed to service the population. So a person living in North Dallas will have plenty of competent surgeons to choose from. The same cannot be said for rural communities or cities that are less desirable to live in. Those areas may not only have a limited supply of surgeons, but the level of expertise and care may be lower than that found in major cities.

That is why managed care organizations are beginning to steer patients needing complex surgery to centers of excellence that may require the person to travel there by car or plane. These large purchasers of care have learned that it is more economical in the long run to refer the person to the best experts and have the surgery done right the first time.

How can you as a consumer locate the best surgeon for your particular problem? There is a logical process that you can follow, and the factors you should consider are discussed in the rest of this chapter.

Choosing a hospital

The key to your outcome will be your surgeon. You can start your search for this person by calling the largest and most prestigious hospital systems in your region because chances are good that the kind of surgeon you are looking for will be on staff at these hospitals. Because these doctors receive complex patients, they will typically do their surgeries at the best hospitals in the area. These hospitals will not only have the intensive care capabilities but also the special surgical instrumentation needed by the spine surgeon.

Remember, though, that a hospital doesn't do your back surgery, a surgeon does. Going to a hospital that performs a large number of back surgeries, only to have a nonspecialized surgeon do your surgery, negates the benefits of going there.

These days a simple back surgery patient will only spend a day or so in the hospital. In some cases a spine surgeon may even do a simple back surgery on an outpatient basis. Where hospital care comes into play is in more complex surgeries requiring instrumentation, or when the person's age or health requires more intensive care resources and back up capabilities if something goes wrong.

Checking out a doctor's record

In many states you can check a physician's record by calling the state medical licensing board. You will find out where the doctor went to school, if the doctor is board-certified, and if any actions have been taken against the doctor's license. You can verify they are board-certified by calling the American Board of Medical Specialties at 1-800-776-2378.

A sad fact is that doctors really don't do a good job of policing themselves. That has caused others, including managed care providers and the government, to start doing the job for them. Massachusetts was one of the first states to pass legislation, in 1996, that gave consumers access to background information on the doctors in that state, including their malpractice histories. The Florida legislature passed a law in May 1997 that will provide doctor profiles to consumers by phone and over the Internet. This program, once approved by the governor, could be running by 1999. Similar bills are pending in California, Connecticut, Illinois, Maine, Maryland, Rhode Island, Texas, and Vermont.

This represents a healthy new consumerism in medicine. Administrators In Medicine (AIM) launched a web site in 1997 at www.docboard.org which contains information on doctors, including "disciplinary actions" but not malpractice histories. In the first four days, the site had 127,000 hits.

Right now, the site only covers Arizona, California, North Carolina, Iowa, Maine, Texas and Vermont. Eventually, the group hopes to have doctor data from all 50 states. More laws are coming that will make malpractice data available as well, something that has been closely guarded by doctors.

Check the certification and level of training Board certification indicates that doctors have measured up to the high standards of their specific board of specialization and to a review by their peers. Board certification is considered by managed care entities and other experts to be a minimum standard for demonstrating clinical expertise in a particular field of medicine.

In most large cities, managed care organizations use board certification to screen and eliminate some physicians from their provider network. For specialists in complex areas, however, they may go more in depth, looking at complication rates, mortality rates, infection rates, length of stay in the hospital, and complexity of patients treated in determining who are the best specialists.

The highest level of training available in orthopedic spine surgery is fellowship. This typically means that the physician has spent a year working at a spine specialty center seeing complex spine patients with senior spine experts. By spending 100 percent of the year focusing on the spine, treating and doing surgery on far more complex patients in that year than the general orthopedic surgeon or neurosurgeon may see over five years, this spine surgeon becomes extremely proficient in spine care. This fellowship training program typically relates to orthopedic surgeons rather than neurosurgeons, who may split their training between spine and brain surgery.

Neurosurgeons vs. orthopedic surgeons

Generally, neurosurgeons perform surgery involving the brain, spinal cord, and other nerves. The specialty of orthopedics focuses on the nonsurgical and surgical treatment of injuries to the musculoskeletal system: the bones, joints, ligaments, muscles, and related nerves, including the spinal cord.

Physicians in both fields begin as medical doctors (M.D.s) or doctors of osteopathy (D.O.s), having completed four years of medical school after finishing their undergraduate degrees. Orthopedic surgeons and neurosurgeons typically spend about one year as interns and then complete five-year residency programs working at a hospital in their respective fields. Next comes board certification. Both orthopedic surgery and neurosurgery have specialty boards that award certification based on written and oral exams as well as the doctor's experience in treating patients.

If you need spine surgery, and are searching for the best surgeon possible, be prepared to hear a lot of criticism volleyed by neurosurgeons at orthopedic surgeons and vice versa. Both will argue that spine surgery is their domain and shouldn't be done by the other specialty. Some of that bias originates in their respective training programs and closely-held beliefs and philosophies. At the risk of oversimplification, the argument centers on the belief that orthopedic surgeons should focus on "bones" while neurosurgeons should focus on "nerves," and therein lies the debate. When a person needs spine surgery, is it because the problem relates to the bones in the spine, or the complicated network of nerves and discs in the spinal column?

Orthopedic surgeons may argue that the bones in the spine may need stabilization to prevent them from moving and causing further damage. This stabilization may be provided by fusing a bone graft between the two vertebrae, or by implanting metal rods or screws that stabilize the spine. Neurosurgeons may argue that some orthopedic surgeons may emphasize screws, plates, rods, and bone grafts in back surgery.

There are excellent spine centers across the United States, some of them founded by orthopedic spine surgeons and some founded by neurosurgeons. Often, they provide the best of both worlds because they use a multi-disciplinary approach that involves both orthopedic surgeons and neurosurgeons. So you can be assured of the best technician for your type of back problem. Managed care organizations in many cities will often contract with both specialties to do back surgery.

Discussing your case

Most physicians understand and respect a patient's desire to receive the best and safest care available. If your doctor won't take the time to fully explain your treatment options and answer your questions, find another specialist.

Getting a second opinion

Many managed care organizations have given up on second opinions, mainly because the physician community too often closes ranks and the second doctor feels a political responsibility to agree with the recommendations of the first.

If you pursue a second opinion, avoid mentioning the conclusions of the first doctor, although this may be difficult because you may be bringing diagnostic studies from the first physician. At least try to select your own second-opinion specialist, rather than taking a recommendation from the first doctor which may be a pass along to an associate who will readily agree.

Case in point: When Pulitzer Prize-winning author Gregory White Smith was told he had a brain tumor and had six months to live, his first reaction was despair. Next, he pursued a second opinion, which only confirmed the first. Then a third, and so on, until he stumbled upon an experimental treatment that arrested the tumor. That was 11 years ago. While he still has the tumor today, medicine has changed over that period and newer treatments hold even more hope that he may continue to survive. Smith put what he has learned into a book called *Making Miracles Happen,* which notes that to get the most out of the health care system consumers must aggressively seek the best medical care, study and explore their options, and decide upon their own best treatment plans.

Some quick tips for evaluating physicians

Most treatments for back problems — even surgical procedures — are elective. This fact gives you time to talk with several specialists to select the physician whose treatment philosophy and qualifications feel most appropriate to you.

When evaluating spine physicians, especially when surgery has been recommended, keep the following in mind:

1. If you need treatment for a serious spine problem, especially one that you suspect might require surgery, seek a "super specialist" — a physician who treats only spine problems and who stays informed and involved in the latest spine research.

This may require an out-of-town trip to a spine center of excellence.

2. View surgery as a last resort. Make sure you and your doctor have given nonsurgical treatments, especially active rehabilitation, every chance to work first.

3. If surgery is recommended, get a second opinion. Any reputable surgeon will respect and even encourage that idea, and many managed care plans reimburse for the expense.

4. Talk to other patients. A good surgeon can provide names of past patients who have undergone the same procedure and may be consulted about what to expect.

5. Make sure you understand your role. Remember, a good spine physician should encourage you to take responsibility for your own recovery with his or her guidance. A full program of postsurgical rehabilitation should be explained to you before you enter the hospital.

6. Make sure your surgeon has a conservative philosophy. A large physical therapy staff can indicate an emphasis on nonsurgical treatment, or at least on good rehabilitation after surgery. The absence of a therapy staff can reflect overreliance on surgery.

7. Finally, check out your surgeon's credentials.

A few questions to ask the doctor

- How long have you been performing this type of surgery, and how many of these operations do you currently perform annually?

  Experience breeds competence, and chances are that a surgeon who performs back surgery regularly keeps up with the latest research into improvements in technique.

- Are you board certified?

  Medical specialists must take tests to become certified by their board of specialty, such as the American Board of Orthopedic Surgery or the American Board of Neurological Surgery.

- What training have you had to perform this surgery?

  Many spine specialists have completed fellowship training, the highest level of schooling in a medical specialty.

CHAPTER 11

What to Do With Pain That Won't Go Away

In physician vernacular, there are two types of pain — acute and chronic. Acute pain is sudden, may come out of nowhere, and be severe and piercing in nature. It serves as a warning signal from the body that something is wrong. The good news is that acute pain eventually will resolve itself when the danger has passed and the cause has been treated. Acute pain serves a useful purpose: it warns us not to continue some activity that is hurting the body.

Then there is chronic pain. The reason this chapter is toward the end of the book is that chronic pain relates only to those people whose back pain has not been relieved with all the mainstream and alternative treatments. Technically speaking, any pain that lasts longer than six months can be categorized as chronic pain. Chronic pain doesn't serve any useful biological purpose. Also, a physician may not be able to find an obvious physical cause for the pain. In other words, chronic pain can be a puzzling medical problem.

The other piece of bad news is that chronic pain can often be the *result* of back surgery — one of the nastier side-effects of becoming a failed back. Consequently, chronic pain sufferers tend to doctor-shop, going from one specialist to another, collecting expensive diagnostic tests and evaluations along the way. The pain condition becomes the predominant focus of the patient and family. Because pain limits a person's activity, sometimes chronic pain sufferers gain weight and get out-of-shape, which causes more complications down the road.

How widespread is chronic pain? It is estimated that 34 million people in the United States suffer from chronic pain of some sort. One researcher estimates that 8 percent of adults in the United States have some sort of persistent pain,[1] and about 2 percent of the U.S. population is estimated to be disabled by chronic back pain. The medical costs for just back pain, headache, and arthritis are pegged at $40 billion annually, and it is estimated that chronic pain accounts for one of every four sick days taken off from work.[2]

Based on a 1997 study by Louis Harris & Associates that surveyed 500 Americans over the age of 60, the National Council of Aging has extrapolated that 18% of elderly Americans regularly take medication for pain that lasts six months or more. Arthritis, joint pain, and lower back pain are the most frequent reasons older Americans are taking drugs. The most popular medications taken are Acetaminophen (Tylenol) 45 percent, and anti-inflammatories (NSAIDS) 39 percent.

Chronic back pain may be sharp, radiating, aching, localized, or diffuse. Chronic muscle pain can include cramping, spasms, stiffness, and swelling. Chronic joint pain can include restricted motion, radiating pain, or heat sensations. Chronic pain may be excruciating or mild, intermittent or continuous, bearable or incapacitating.

Finding the source of chronic pain and treating it properly can be complicated, to say the least. Some physicians run for cover when they hear a patient complain of chronic pain, because they know from experience that chronic pain is frustrating to treat.

Some chronic pain sufferers feel that physicians view them as crazy. That's because physicians are not able to measure pain, and if they find no physiological cause, some may believe that it's all in the patient's head. That just adds to the frustration of the chronic pain sufferer whose life becomes an endless, frustrating search for relief.

The first step in resolving chronic pain from back or neck injury is to try to find out exactly what is causing the pain signal to the brain. This is like trying to sort out a massive short circuit after lightning hits your fusebox. The unfortunate reality is that nearly 80 percent of all back pain sufferers will never learn the exact cause of their pain.

Even if a physical cause is identified and treated, by the time this happens the chronic pain may have taken on an additional psychological dimension — almost like a Twilight Zone of chronic pain. This psychological dimension can confound treatment.

For some patients who have back and neck surgery for a relatively simple disc problem, only to wake up with something much worse, one immediate thought is, "Well, let's do surgery again — and get it right this time." Unfortunately, while the initial surgery may have removed the herniated disc, during the process a nerve may have been damaged, and no additional surgery can fix a damaged nerve. The only option left involves blocking the pain coming from the damaged nerve. This again is why surgery should always be the last resort. Even if something is simple, and the surgery "appears" to go well, nerves may be affected in the process of cutting.

The difficulty of treating something you can't see

No two people experience pain the same way or find relief in the same way. One person may experience agony from a particular injury while another complains of only minor discomfort.

Perception is an important factor in the study and treatment of pain. The pain signal from an injury travels along a series of nerve fibers to the brain. There are numerous ways the pain message may be altered or even canceled along the route.

The body has the ability to produce chemicals called endorphins, which act as natural drugs to dull the perception of pain. These endorphins act by attaching themselves to certain receptors in the brain and throughout the body. How can you turn on the body's own drug manufacturing center? Emotions can do it, so can meditation and acupuncture. What is even more relevant is that exercise is known to stimulate the brain to produce endorphins.

Another non-narcotic pain-relieving technique is biofeedback. A person in pain naturally tends to tighten the muscles that surround the painful area in an unconscious attempt to protect the site of injury. Tension can increase pain, which in turn generates more tension. With practice, patients who have been taught biofeedback techniques can release tension and break the pain-tension cycle.

Treating chronic pain

There is hope for chronic pain sufferers. In the last five years, there has been a high volume of research literature focusing on pain management, and there are multi-disciplinary pain centers starting up that specialize in this complex problem.

Chronic pain is treated in a lot of different ways by a lot of different people. In an effort to standardize chronic pain treatment, the U.S. Government's Agency for Health Care Policy and Research (AHCPR) has developed clinical guidelines for pain management directed at pain care providers.

One survey of 263 pain treatment centers tried to identify how pain is currently treated and what treatments appear to work best. The treatments most commonly used by therapists at these pain clinics were individualized exercise programs, relaxation training, TENS, training in body mechanics, and biofeedback.[3] Similarly, an analysis of 76 research studies on treatment of chronic back pain yielded strong evidence that certain medications, limited use of chiropractic manipulation, back schools, and exercise are effective.[4]

As we have previously noted, while a physician can prescribe heavy narcotics to relieve pain "symptoms," this is not a good treatment because many drugs have complicated side effects that, with prolonged use, can damage internal organs. There is also the possibility of addiction, which creates an entirely new problem in itself.

Spine centers that treat a lot of chronic pain often receive patients who have been treated with an array of pain medications used to mask the source of pain. But to get to the root of the problem and develop a treatment plan that isn't dependent upon drugs often requires a detox step, to remove the person from their drug dependency.

Fortunately, there are ways to help patients with chronic pain who are completely dependent on drugs. For example, the patient and family members may be able to talk about the pain and their complex feelings with a psychologist specializing in chronic pain. These professionals can help patients find ways of overcoming emotional conditions and stress, and they can play a key role in sorting out the "real reason" someone may not be getting better with medical treatment. Psychologists and therapists can also help patients learn to control their pain without extended reliance on habit-forming drugs.

Some managed care companies are suspicious of psychologists working with pain patients. This concern may not be warranted. Any approach that gets the patient back to work and activity sooner will save money in disability claims and lost productivity.

Chronic pain can also cause a second problem: depression. No surprise; after living with pain for months and years, what normal person wouldn't get depressed? But the long-term effect is that depression — accompanied by anxiety, stress, anger, and fatigue — inhibits the body's ability to manufacture pain-killing endorphins. Then the cycle gets continually worse. It is also easy for a chronic pain sufferer to slip from an active life to a sedentary one. Consequently, a person may become deconditioned and gain weight, making recovery even more difficult. Extended periods of disability and time away from work also restrict income, create worry, and decrease a person's feelings of self-worth. This may further isolate the patient from co-workers, friends, and even family members, who may be frustrated as well.

Next, the body's own immune defenses get weakened by all the above, which in turn makes the chronic pain sufferer vulnerable to other illnesses. The process of recovery from long-term chronic pain is like crawling out of a deep abyss.

Pain clinics

Pain clinics are relatively new in the health care industry. Currently, there are about 1,500 such clinics or centers across the country, focusing solely on the treatment of chronic pain. They may be associated with a hospital or may be operated by anesthesiologists who specialize in treating pain.

At their worst, some pain clinics are viewed as "shot depots," where anesthesiologists merely administer more and more injections to mask pain. The best and most respected pain clinics, however, use a multi-disciplinary approach to pain involving physicians, psychologists, physical therapists, and alternative healers.

Physical Therapy Chronic pain patients are often in poor physical condition because they fear activity and exercise will make them worse. Studies suggest the opposite is true. Activity is the key to physical conditioning and mental outlook. It is common for long-term back and neck pain sufferers to have back stiffness and weakness, which can be helped with physical therapy. A program of regular stretching, strengthening, and physical conditioning exercises is an important part of chronic pain rehabilitation. These activities are led by a physical therapist with an interest in chronic pain conditions.

Functional Rehabilitation By simulating the activities of daily living or activities done at work, an occupational therapist can make recovery and therapy more "practical" or "functional." Therapists will show the patient safe ways to lift, bend, and twist, and to perform work-related duties. A return to functional activity is the first step in helping the individual feel less like a victim and more like a productive person. Getting back to work can improve one's mood and create challenges that may distract the mind from pain.

Medication Management It is becoming more acceptable for doctors to provide narcotics to patients suffering from chronic pain. Still, doctors need to be very concerned about the risk of physical dependence and addiction. Long term, sorting out a person's pain problem may begin with needing to detox the patient. The physician may also prescribe medications such as nonsteroidal anti-inflammatory agents (NSAIDS) and tricyclic anti-depressants to decrease the dose of narcotics needed to make the patients comfortable.

Relaxation Training Relaxation training can be a valuable skill for any person experiencing back or neck pain. It helps patients learn to modify the tension associated with their chronic pain condition and break the pain-tension cycle. Learning to relax can be a powerful tool in combating chronic pain, and helps the patient to take responsibility for treating their pain condition.

Centers that work with chronic back and neck pain sufferers often use a certified biofeedback technician. While biofeedback was not initially developed as a treatment for chronic pain, many clinicians now regard it as the treatment of choice for a variety of pain syndromes, especially lower back pain. One of the rationales for the use of biofeedback is that it can be used to modify the specific physiological processes that are believed to underlie the pain disorder. Biofeedback equipment uses low-level electrical impulses to translate muscle tension into audible signals. With the aid of a biofeedback expert the patient is taught to relax affected muscles, which in turn changes the audible signal.

Guided imagery techniques can sometimes achieve similar results without the equipment. Here are some basic guidelines for starting the process simply. Done correctly, these techniques can interrupt one's present focus on pain and start the healing process. Here are some simple relaxation and guided imagery steps:

1. Find a quiet place and a comfortable position. If you are wearing a tie, loosen it. If you are at home, this exercise can be done in a warm bath.

2. Give yourself a full 30 minutes to relax. Don't skip this step; you may sabotage your relaxation. Give yourself permission to take the time to relax. Tell yourself that you have no place to go, nothing else to do that is more important. Commit to spending the entire time on your relaxation exercise.

3. Focus on your breathing. Slowly close your eyes and take slow deep breaths. Concentrate on how your chest rises and falls with each slow breath. Imagine that with each breath you are discharging more and more tension.

4. Imagine yourself in a desirable, relaxing setting, maybe a warm, sunny beach. Challenge your imagination to duplicate what you would be hearing, seeing, smelling, or touching on that beach. Try to feel the heat of the sun on your skin. Try to remember what suntan lotion smells like. Imagine your hands stroking the sand and try to feel the texture. What else can you see on that beach? Are there others around? What are they wearing?

Another relaxation technique is called "progressive relaxation," where you systematically tense each muscle from your toes to your head for a few seconds, and then relax it. Researchers have determined that a muscle relaxes much more if it is tensed completely first.

Nerve blocks and injections Injections in the spine have a dual purpose: they provide relief from pain, and they help the doctor determine the source of pain. For example, an anesthesiologist may administer several injections to determine the precise level in the spine that may be causing pain. Once the diagnosis is made, a dose of steroid — a potent anti-inflammatory agent — can be injected near the pain generator, which may be an irritated nerve root in the spine or in the facet joints of the back.

Various injection treatments reduce inflammation and pain by blocking the nerve impulses carrying the pain message. These blocks can help reduce postural stress and allow the person to participate in exercise and other rehabilitation.

Generally, with chronic back and neck pain, there are three types of injections: epidural steroid, facet joint, and trigger point. Epidural steroid injection therapy is believed to be helpful in cases of sciatica, where a steroid is injected into the epidural space surrounding the spinal cord and nerves.

Facet joints, when they work properly, enable spinal bones to glide over each other while the back is in motion. Over time, due to many factors, these joints can become painful. An injection may be given directly into the joint to relieve this pain. Trigger point injections actually anesthetize the point of pain in a muscle or at another location that may be transmitting the pain signal.

All three of these injections produce temporary relief of pain. They are most effective when combined with other treatments and should only be used as a part of a comprehensive treatment plan.

Sometimes longer-acting techniques are used, such as freezing the painful nerve (cryoneurolysis) or heating the nerve with radio frequency. While the effects of these treatments last longer, they also do not offer a permanent cure.

Using electricity to block pain Some patients may wear TENS (Transcutaneous Electrical Nerve Stimulation) units to temporarily interrupt pain signals to the brain. Although there is some debate about exactly how TENS works, proponents argue that the intermittent electrical current causes the brain to release endorphins, the body's natural painkillers. Some research maintains that the use of TENS does not significantly improve clinical outcomes.

Long-term severe pain sufferers may even consider suicide as the only real escape. For those extreme cases, doctors may recommend such extreme measures as implanting a small electrical stimulator in the spine. This type of surgery is based on the Gate Control theory of pain. This theory states that any sensation — a touch, a pinprick, a tickle — travels by electrical impulses through the spinal cord to the brain, and that an electrical signal can turn off or close the "pain gate" so the brain is unable to receive the pain signal.

In a procedure called Spinal Cord Stimulation, electrodes are placed near the area in the spine that is thought to be transmitting the pain signal to the brain. Using an external device the size of a hand-held radio, the physician can program the implanted electrical stimulator to send a tiny electrical signal at the precise intervals when the pain site is cycling out pain messages. The result is that the signals cancel each other out, leaving a slight tingling sensation. Spinal cord stimulators also stimulate the brain and spinal cord to secrete a substance that helps to reduce pain. This explains why there is a prolonged analgesic effect even after the unit is turned off.

Spinal cord stimulation, traditionally, is only appropriate for certain types of pain. With the advent of dual lead stimulators we are now able to provide pain relief for patients with lumbar as well as leg pain. The technology can also be used for neck and arm pain.

Spinal cord stimulators have been used since the 1970s. Over the years the technique and the technology have continually improved, with the implanted units becoming smaller and the electrical signal becoming more controlled and effective. It is estimated that about 50,000 patients worldwide have had spinal cord stimulators implanted.

The chief benefit of a spinal cord stimulator is that pain relief is achieved with a small electrical current applied to the spinal cord instead of by injecting potentially harmful drugs into the body. Implanting a spinal cord stimulator also doesn't burn any bridges. If the treatment doesn't work the stimulator can be removed, and there are typically no permanent complications.

Because of the large number of complex failed back patients referred there, spinal cord stimulators have been used for several years by Dr. Ralph Rashbaum at the Texas Back Institute. A follow-up study of spinal cord stimulator patients two years after implant showed that 70 percent would recommend the stimulator to a friend with a similar problem. Another 84 percent noted that they had decreased or eliminated their use of narcotics.[5]

Implantable drug pumps In other extreme cases, a physician may consider the implantation of a morphine pump, a device which trickles medication into the spinal fluid. The advantage of this method over taking a drug orally is that a precise level of medication is provided at a fraction of the dosage and with a more even flow than if the medication were injected or taken orally. For someone who would have to take drugs orally for the long term, an implanted pump is probably a better option. The smaller dosage needed translates into a cost savings as well. For example, the dose of morphine used through a pump is 1/300th the dose of morphine that would be taken by mouth. Also, pain relief is often better with the pump delivery system.

Such implantable pumps have been used since the 1980s for chemotherapy, and morphine pumps have been in use since 1991. It is estimated that about 25,000 people worldwide have had drug pumps implanted.

Patients with extreme symptoms present ethical dilemmas for the treating physician. One physician may feel that providing pain-relieving narcotics is counterproductive in the long term and can damage internal organs further. Another physician may observe the pain and suffering of the individual and feel the most compassionate route is to prescribe drugs that can provide relief, albeit temporary. The latter approach poses additional problems because a physician may risk losing her or his license if accused of prescribing narcotics too liberally.

Who is appropriate for a pain clinic Pain clinics should be considered only after a medical doctor has performed a thorough examination to rule out any and all physical causes of pain such as a tumor. Pain clinic staff should be sensitive to the effect of the pain on all aspects of the patient's life. Patients are often focused on the short-term relief derived from drugs or injections, and physicians must gear their thinking to long-term pain management.

As we stated early on in the book, 80 percent of back pain will go away on its own. Most of the other 20 percent will get relief over time with the help of physicians and therapists. A small percentage of people, probably less than one percent of back and neck pain sufferers, may have to deal with ongoing back or neck pain for the rest of their lives.

The intent of the pain treatment provider is to change the patient's focus from what they *can't* do because of pain to what activities of daily life they *can* do, and how to improve on those. The name of the game is focusing on function, not pain. By getting people moving again, and enabling them to walk, drive, work, even exercise, their minds can move out of the focus of pain, and the body's endorphins can begin to play a supporting role again.

People with chronic back and neck pain should try to find pastimes that can distract their minds from pain, whether those pastimes involve physical activity or not. Painting, flower arranging, fishing, photography, and even watching children or grandchildren play sports are a few ideas for those who cannot tolerate much physical activity. If you can move, walking or light gardening can get you out of the house and improve your mood. The more physical movement you can bring back into your life, the easier it is for healing to begin. Time spent with family and friends will also help you feel better and will give those who care about you some encouragement that you aren't throwing in the towel. Try not to use time with others to complain about your pain, which serves only to focus on it.

What to look for in a pain clinic The director of a pain clinic should be board certified in anesthesiology, physical medicine and rehabilitation, or psychology, and also in pain management. A good pain clinic will use a multi-disciplinary approach in diagnosis and treatment, with staff that could include a clinical psychologist, anesthesiologist, physical therapist, registered nurse, certified biofeedback therapist, vocational counselor, nutritionist, social worker, occupational therapist, massage therapist, and acupuncturist or chiropractor. They should all meet together frequently to discuss diagnoses and treatment plans for all patients admitted to the pain clinic.

The American Academy of Pain Management (AAPM) and the Commission on Accreditation of Rehabilitation Facilities (CARF) have been surveying and accrediting pain management programs across the country. AAPM can be reached at 209-533-9744 and CARF can be reached at 520-325-1044. Both organizations can provide a list of accredited clinics.

Pain clinics can be extremely expensive because of all the diagnostic tests and treatments involved. This expense is one reason many managed care organizations view them with suspicion. Some managed care organizations will audit the functional status of a pain sufferer before they enter the clinic by asking if they can climb stairs, carry groceries, do their job, etc. Then after diagnostics and treatment at a pain clinic, the patient completes a second questionnaire. Unfortunately, while the pain patients may find some relief, too often there is no "measurable" improvement as far as the managed care organization is concerned. Because they are the ones paying the bills, they are extremely cautious about referrals to pain clinics.

This has put great pressure on those in the pain field to produce definable positive outcomes. The best pain clinics are making progress in this regard, designing protocols that specify clear and understandable treatment pathways, and winning back the confidence of referring physicians.

Notes

1. Von Korff, M., Wagner, E., Dworkin, S., et al. "Chronic Pain and the Use of Ambulatory Health Care." *Psychosomatic Medicine* 53 (1991): 61–79.
2. *US News & World Report* (March 17, 1997).
3. Doliber, C.M. "Role of the Physical Therapist at Pain Treatment Centers. A Survey." *Physical Therapy* 64 (1984): 905–909.
4. Van Tulder, M.W., Koes, B.W., Bouter, L.M. "Conservative Treatment of Acute and Chronic Nonspecific Low Back Pain." *Spine* 22 no. 18 (1997): 2128–2156.
5. Ohnmeiss, D., Rashbaum, R., Bogdanffy, G. *Spine* 21 (1996):1344–1351.

CHAPTER 12

Back to the Future

The next few years may prove to be a period of great change in how back problems are treated, thanks to new research involving non-surgical treatment alternatives. Researchers are trying to find out what is the best way to resolve back and neck pain, and are asking why certain countries like the United States are so quick to resort to the knife when it comes to treating back pain.

Employers and managed care organizations are driving this change, by challenging the traditional enthusiasm of surgeons to rush into back surgery. Managed care companies and large employers around the United States already have their own studies underway to see what is the best and most cost effective way to treat various back problems. Several managed care companies, like Blue Cross in Georgia, Aetna/US Healthcare in Maryland, PacifiCare in California, and Cigna in Tennessee, all have panels of physicians working to develop back care clinical protocols for physicians who want to see patients from these companies.

Some employers and managed care organizations have also mandated second opinions to stop unnecessary spine surgeries. Others are steering their employees away from surgeons and toward non-surgeon "gatekeepers" like primary care physicians and physical medicine and rehabilitation (PMR) physicians. Others are mandating that physicians follow non-surgical clinical protocols.

For example, in Memphis, Tennessee, where FedEx is headquartered with its thousands of employees who lift boxes, Cigna and FedEx have worked together to improve how back care is provided, and a part of that process was developing clinical protocols to improve quality.

The age of the enlightened consumer

Many back problems get better on their own. In most cases surgery can be delayed, allowing the pain symptoms to disappear. Even if surgery is ultimately necessary, the knowledgeable consumer can do a great deal to increase his or her chances of a successful spine surgery. Even if you don't have a managed care company or employer asking concerned questions about your spine treatment, *you* should ask questions. Most spine experts do not have a problem with questions. In fact, they encourage them.

Today, a new consumerism is cutting across all areas of health care. Beginning in 1997, the National Library of Medicine made Medline, a compendium of 9 million references and abstracts from 4,000 medical journals previously limited to the medical community, available free to consumers via the Internet. The response? Within two months, the Medline web site was logging one million visits a day.

This is creating a new industry: companies that research the latest treatments for complex diseases, not for doctors, but for consumers who want to know more about their problems.

Are informed consumers better off? A 1994 study by Harvard University's School of Public Health showed that fully informed consumers usually choose less risky and less expensive options than do those with little information.

If and when you end up needing to see a doctor, use all the information in this book to make yourself an informed consumer. Research new treatments on the Internet. Find the best spine specialist in your area who emphasizes non-surgical cures rather than surgery. Or find a spine specialty clinic with all the best possible non-surgical treatments under one roof. Remember, unless you have emergency symptoms that require immediate surgery, you can delay back surgery — if you can tolerate the pain. Long term outcome studies show that after a couple of years you can't tell the difference between those who were treated with surgery and those who skipped surgery in favor of non-surgical care.

Lastly, ask questions, and lots of them. If your physician has a problem with you wanting to understand your care, that's a sure sign you need to find another doctor who is interested in you playing an active role in your recovery and maintaining your own health. Taking responsibility for your health is the first important step back toward a healthy, active life. We hope the information in this book plays a part in getting you there.

Resources

Checking out a healthcare provider's record

You can check a physician's record in many states by calling the state medical licensing board. You will find out where the doctor went to school, if the doctor is board-certified and if any actions have been taken against the doctor's license. You can verify if the doctor is board-certified by calling the American Board of Medical Specialties at 1-800-776-2378.

Biofeedback therapists are licensed by the Association for Applied Psychophysiology and Biofeedback (AAPB). The AAPB can be reached at 1-800-477-8892 for information on biofeedback experts in your area.

Resources if you are suffering from chronic pain

The Worldwide Congress on Pain
http://www.pain.com

WellnessWeb
http://www.wellweb.com

National Chronic Pain Outreach Association 540-997-5004

American Academy of Pain Management (AAPM) 209-533-9744

Information and support organizations

Alexander Technique Society 1-800-473-0620

American Academy of Physical Medicine & Rehabilitation 312-464-9700

American Association of Naturopathic Physicians 206-323-7610

American Board of Medical Specialties 1-800-776-2378

American Massage Therapy Assocation 708-864-0123

American Osteopathic Association 1-800-621-1773

Arthritis Foundation 1-800-283-7800

Association for Applied Psychophysiology & Biofeedback (AAPB) 1-800-477-8892

Aston Patterning 702-831-8228

Ayurvedic Institute 505-291-9698

Commission on Accreditation of Rehabilitation Facilities (CARF) 520-325-1044

Feldenkrais Association 1-800-775-2118

International Assocation of Yoga Therapists 415-383-4587

National Acupuncture and Oriental Medicine Alliance . . 206-524-3511

National Certification Commission for Acupuncture & Oriental Medicine 202-232-1404

National Osteoporosis Foundation 1-800-223-9994

Reflexology Institute 813-343-4811

Rolf Institute 1-800-530-8875

Scoliosis Association 1-800-800-0669

Nurse staffed information lines

Texas Back Institute, Plano, Texas . . . . 1-800-247-BACK(2225)

Mayfield Spine Institute, Cincinnati, Ohio 1-800-696-BACK

Center for Spine, Savannah, Georgia 1-912-691-BACK

Resources to explore on the Internet

The top four . . .

National Library of Medicine
http://www.nlm.nih.gov
This is the ultimate source on the Internet for health information. It provides access to its Grateful Med database which includes Medline (see below) and thousands of links to health information on the Internet.

MEDLINE
http://www.nlm.nih.gov/databases/medline.html
A database of more than 8.8 million references to articles published in 3,800 biomedical journals.

National Institutes of Health
http://www.nih.gov
Gives hyperlinks to all of the organizations that make up the National Institutes of Health.

National Institutes of Health Office of Alternative Medicine
http://altmed.od.nih.gov/oam
The National Institutes of Health's Office of Alternative Medicine (OAM) was created in 1991 to identify and evaluate helpful cures for a variety of health problems. The OAM's web site has a frequently asked questions section and subsections on various health problems and alternative medicine solutions.

. . . and many more

Achoo Online Health Services
http://www.achoo.com
This site connects visitors to thousands of health care sites. It also provides a list of news groups, headline health news categorized into more than 150 topics, and a site of the week.

Alternative Medicine
http://www.pitt.edu/~cbw/altm.html
This site describes itself as "a jump station for information on unconventional, unorthodox, unproven, or alternative, complimentary, innovative, integrated therapies."

Agency for Health Care Policy and Research (AHCPR)
http://www.ahcpr.gov
Offers thousands of free publication through snail mail or to download through the web site. Publications cover every major health-related topic with versions for health care providers and patients.

American Medical Association Doctor Finder
http://www.ama-assn.org/
Allows visitors to search a database for doctors in their area.

Chiro Web
http://pages.prodigy.com/CT/doc/doc.html
Provides information and links to chiropractic resources on the Internet. The site also covers basic information such as licensing, research, associations, etc.

Combined Health Information Index
http://chid.nih.gov
Provides titles, abstracts, and availability information for health education resources from all over the world.

Family Medicine Related Internet Resources
http://griffin.vcu.edu/views.vcu.edu/-dim list/
The North American Primary Care Research Group provides general health information and hyperlinks to health organizations and associations, university family practice programs, hospitals, e-mail lists, nursing and educational materials.

Food & Drug Administration
http://www.fda.gov

Health Hotlines
http://sis.nlm.nih.gov/hotlines
The National Library of Medicine offers this online database of health related organizations operating toll-free telephone services. The database also includes information services and publications in Spanish.

Health World Online
http://www.healthy.net
This site allows visitors to browse volumes of health information on a wide variety of topics. It provides legislative and news information along with a venue for participating in health forums or to ask Dr. Tom a question.

HSTAT — Health Services/Technology Assessment Text
http://text.nlm.nih.gov
An electronic resource that includes full text versions of clinical practice guidelines, quick reference guides for clinicians, and consumer brochures.

Medical Matrix
http://www.kumc.edu:80/mmatrix
This database offers access to thousands of health related articles, journals, publications, etc.

Medscape
http://www.medscape.com
This site is geared toward health care professionals and medical students. It contains original, full text medical articles which tend to be highly technical.

Medsite
http://www.medsite.com
This site promotes itself as "your online source for medical information." Medsite acts as a medical search engine for health care topics, and will provide links to Medline, Medchat, Medlink, and press releases in the health care arena.

Multimedia Medical Reference Library
http://www.med-library.com
This site offers links to hundreds of health-related sources on the Internet.

National Health Information Center
http://nhic-nt.health.org
This site puts health professionals, organizations, and consumers in touch with each other. Its database includes more than 1,000 organizations and government agencies that provide health information.

New England Journal of Medicine
http://www.nejm.org
This site serves as an online version of the New England Journal of Medicine that offers access to back issues and links to other health care related sites on the Internet.

Reuters Health Information Services
http://www.reutershealth.com
This site allows visitors to search health news headlines and access full stories from its vast news archives. The site is geared toward health professionals and contains links to many other health related sites on the Internet.

Choosing a hospital

US News Online: America's Best Hospitals
http://www4.usnews.com/usnews/nycu/hosphigh.htm
This site ranks America's hospitals on quality of care in several categories. For a specific listing of neurological hospitals go to http://www4.usnews.com/usnews/nycu/neurolog.htm.

Choosing a doctor

http://www.lhs-be-well.org/

This comprehensive site includes a list of pre-screening questions you should ask a potential doctor. It provides a list of specialties and their definitions; discusses insurance, HMOs, and PPOs; and gives specific advice on how to communicate with your doctor and what information you should and should not divulge.

DocFinder

http://www.docboard.org

Allows visitors to search by state and name for physician licensing information, credentials, and board certification status.

How to Choose (and get the maximum mileage from) Your Primary Care Doctor

http://www.coolware.com/health/joel/choosing.html

Online Medical Reference System

http://www.kumc.edu/service/dykes/refassist/facts/rankrec.html

This site provides bibliographic information on all types of doctors and dentists across the nation. A literature search is also offered on this site along with many useful address and phone numbers.

Mail Order Sources

Back Be Nimble 1-800-639-3746

Healthy Back Store 1-800-469-2225

Books and publications

Ayurveda: The A-Z Guide to Healing Techniques from Ancient India,
by Helen Thomas, Nancy Pauline Bruning, Island Books, 1997.

Ayurveda: Life Health and Longevity,
by Robert E. Svoboda, Arkana Press, 1993.

Back Care Basics: A Doctor's Gentle Yoga Program for Back and Neck Pain Relief,
by Mary Pullig Schatz,Rodmell Press, 1992.

Back in Balance: A Chronic Pain Workbook,
by Barbara J. Headley, 1998.

Making Miracles Happen,
by Gregory White Smith, Steven W. Naifeh, Little, Brown,1997.

Managing Chronic Pain: Strategies for Dealing with Back Pain, Muscle and Joint Pain, Cancer Pain, Abdominal Pain
by Sian-Yang Tan, Intravarsity Press, 1996.

Mastering Miracles: The Healing Art of Qi Gong as Taught by a Master
by Hong Liu, Paul Perry, Warner Books, 1997.

Qi Gong for Beginners: Eight Easy Movements for Vibrant Health,
by Stanley D. Wilson, Rudra Press, 1997.

Index

N

O

P

Q

R

S

T

V

W

X

Y

About the Authors

Working together over 10 years, Stephen Hochschuler, M.D., and Bob Reznik, MBA, helped develop Texas Back Institute, which was the nation's largest spine specialty clinic in 1995. In that year, more than 10,000 back pain sufferers from around the United States came to the Institute to see the fellowship-trained spine specialists there. Over that 10 year period, the Texas Back Institute was also featured on NBC's "Today Show," "CBS This Morning," and CNN, and in *USA Today, Fortune, Forbes, Good Housekeeping, Woman's Day, Golf, McCall's, Better Homes, Ladies Home Journal,* and many other national media.

The Texas Back Institute operates a free medical information line at 1-800-247-BACK, staffed with nurses who can answer general questions about back pain. As a free community service, the Texas Back Institute also sends out home remedy and home exercise information that enables many people to resolve their own back pain at home. The Institute also has an internet site at www.texasback.com.

About Bob Reznik, MBA

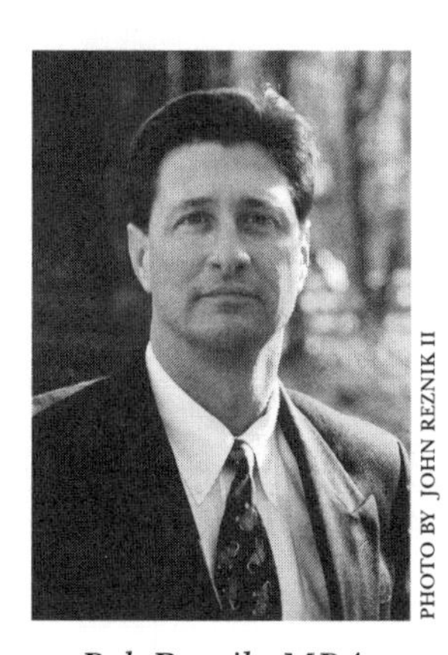

PHOTO BY JOHN REZNIK II

Bob Reznik, MBA

Bob Reznik believes that health care can be improved if people learn to modify their lifestyles to prevent health problems, detect problems early when they occur, and then seek out the best possible doctors for care. Reznik exercises regularly to prevent back injury. So far, his back exercises have enabled him to play golf and tennis competitively without strain.

Reznik's company, Prizm Development, Inc., works with healthcare providers around the United States to develop consumer-friendly centers of excellence in a variety of fields. The protocols and software systems developed by Prizm help physicians reduce treatment variation, and improve how they care for and communicate with the patient. Prizm is based in Grapevine, Texas and can be reached at www.prizmbrochure.com or by e-mail at prizm@flash.net.

About Stephen Hochschuler, M.D.

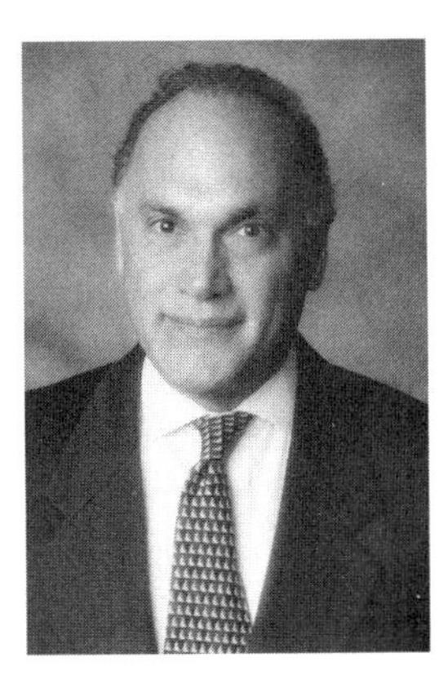

Dr. Stephen Hochschuler

Internationally known, Dr. Stephen Hochschuler is a board-certified orthopedic surgeon who specializes in spine surgery. He received his medical degree from Harvard Medical School in Boston. In 1986, Dr. Hochschuler and two partners, Dr. Ralph Rashbaum and Dr. Richard Guyer, founded Texas Back Institute. Dr. Hochschuler has edited two spine textbooks, *Rehabilitation of the Spine* and *The Spine in Sports*. In 1990, he authored *Back in Shape*, a book for back pain sufferers. Over the past 15 years he has served as a clinical instructor at the University of Texas Southwestern Medical School in the Department of Orthopedics. Dr. Hochschuler is currently Chairman of Texas Back Institute.

Texas Back Institute is based in Plano, a suburb of Dallas, Texas, and has offices across North Texas. Dr. Hochschuler continues to see back patients at Texas Back Institute offices in Dallas, Midland, and Wichita Falls.

As someone who practices what he preaches, he has never had to resort to back surgery for his own back problem. He reduces his risk of occasional back pain attacks by exercising regularly and staying active in many sports, including biking, hiking, and skiing.

HEALTH

MENOPAUSE WITHOUT MEDICINE *by* Linda Ojeda, Ph.D.

Linda Ojeda broke new ground when she began her study of nonmedical approaches to menopause more than ten years ago. In this update of her classic book, she discusses natural sources of estrogen; how mood swings are affected by diet and personality; and the newest research on osteoporosis, breast cancer, and heart disease. She thoroughly examines the hormone therapy debate; suggests natural remedies for depression, hot flashes, sexual changes, and skin and hair problems. **As seen in *Time* magazine.**

352 pages ... 40 illus. ... Paperback $14.95 ... Hard cover $23.95 ... 3rd edition

HER HEALTHY HEART: A Woman's Guide to Preventing and Reversing Heart Disease Naturally *by* Linda Ojeda, Ph.D.

Heart disease is the #1 killer of women. Linda Ojeda, Ph.D., bestselling author of *Menopause Without Medicine*, gives women the facts about this disease and describes ways they can prevent it naturally. She discusses nutrition factors and what women can do to modify their diet to benefit their heart. Individual chapters discuss fat, fiber, protein, B-vitamins, and antioxidants. Finally Ojeda discusses lifestyle changes such as managing stress and taking the time to enjoy life.

356 pages ... 12 illus. ... Paperback $14.95 ... Available September 1998

RUNNING ON EMPTY: The Complete Guide to Chronic Fatigue Syndrome (CFIDS) *by* Katrina Berne, Ph.D.

Sore throat, fatigue, vertigo, headache, muscle pain, fever, depression — if you are unable to shake these symptoms you may be suffering from Chronic Fatigue Syndrome. Although it can be difficult to diagnose, CFIDS is a real, biologically-based disease with options for effective treatment and management. Written by an expert who has CFIDS herself, this book includes summaries of recent medical findings on treatments, ideas on living with the disease, and intimate stories of other sufferers. This is both an invaluable book for CFIDS patients and a complete reference for the health care professionals who treat them.

336 pages ... Paperback $14.95 ... Hard cover $24.95 ... 2nd edition

MACULAR DEGENERATION — AN AGING-EYE DISEASE: A Guide to Recognizing and Controlling Symptoms, Understanding Treatment Options, and Learning to Live Productively with Vision Loss
by Betty Wason and James McMillan, M.D.

Age-related macular degeneration (AMD) is an affliction of progressive vision loss and is the leading cause of legal blindness for people over the age of 50. Betty Wason contracted this eye disease and together with Dr. James McMillan offers readers a complete resource for people with AMD and their families. Topics include: what happens to the eye as a result of AMD, how to choose a doctor, diet and food supplements that can help, high-tech and low-tech products that can help with everyday activities, and the important role of family members.

224 pages ... 10 illus. ... Paperback $13.95 ... Available September 1998

To order books or a FREE catalog see last page or call (800) 266-5592

WOMEN'S HEALTH / NUTRITION

GETTING PREGNANT AND STAYING PREGNANT: Overcoming Infertility and Managing Your High-Risk Pregnancy *by* Diana Raab, R.N.

This is a practical guide to the physical, medical, and emotional issues women and their partners face during infertility treatments and high-risk pregnancies. Winner of the 1992 Benjamin Franklin Award for Best Health Book, it combines accurate medical information with a nurse's thoughtfulness and care. The book covers new infertility technologies, tests, and genetic risks and combines information about what to expect during a high-risk pregnancy with supportive ideas for coping with cesareans, miscarriages, and premature babies.

336 pages ... 28 illus. ... Paperback ... $14.95

THE FERTILITY AWARENESS HANDBOOK: The Natural Guide to Avoiding or Achieving Pregnancy *by* Barbara Kass-Annese, R.N., and Hal C. Danzer, M.D.

The language of a woman's body tells her the days of the month when she is most fertile and likely to conceive, and when she is infertile and can safely have sex without conceiving. The methods described in this book are based on this language and give women a contraceptive choice or an enhanced opportunity to become pregnant. These scientifically proven methods have no side-effects, no hormone-related dangers. They teach women to be more in touch with their bodies, more secure in lovemaking, and more in control of their sexual well-being.

160 pages ... 47 illus. ... Paperback ... $11.95

ONCE A MONTH: The Original Premenstrual Syndrome Handbook *by* Katharina Dalton, M.D.

Once considered an imaginary complaint, PMS has at last received the serious attention it deserves, thanks largely to the work of Dr. Katharina Dalton. Premenstrual syndrome may in fact be the world's most common condition: surveys show that as many as 75% of women experience at least one symptom. The fifth edition of this classic book covers all the issues including the symptoms, effects, and medical and self-help treatment options.

288 pages ... 36 illus. ... Paperback ... $14.95 ... 5th edition

FAD-FREE NUTRITION *by* Fredrick J. Stare, M.D., Ph.D., and Elizabeth M. Whelan, Sc.D., M.P.H.

The media is flooded with claims of quick-fix nutritional nirvanas. Using up-to-date nutrition information and basing their approach on sound scientific principles and legitimate studies, the authors help the reader sort fact from fiction. They debunk claims that the food supply is irreversibly tainted, that disease is an inevitable result of eating, that nutritional supplements are a necessity, and that food technology is employed against the public interest.

Fredrick J. Stare, M.D., Ph.D., founded the Department of Nutrition at Harvard University's School of Public Health in 1942. **Elizabeth M. Whelan, Sc.D., M.P.H.,** is president and a founder of the American Council on Science and Health.

256 pages ... Paperback $14.95 ... Available April 1998

To order books or a FREE catalog see last page or call (800) 266-5592

SEXUALITY

SEXUAL PLEASURE: Reaching New Heights of Sexual Arousal and Intimacy *by* Barbara Keesling, Ph.D.

This book is for everyone interested in enhancing his or her sex life so that lovemaking becomes a deep physical and emotional exchange. It shows how to develop sensual awareness and learn to replace anxiety with enjoyment. A series of graduated sensual exercises reveal the three secrets of sexual pleasure: enjoying touching, enjoying being touched, and merging touching and feeling as an ecstatic experience. Sensual photographs add a note of artistic intimacy and make this book the perfect personal gift for caring partners.

224 pages ... 14 b&w photos ... Paperback $13.95 ... Hard cover $21.95

MAKING LOVE BETTER THAN EVER: Exploring New Ways to Sexual Pleasure *by* Barbara Keesling, Ph.D.

Making Love Better than Ever is for loving couples looking for sexual adventure within their monogamous relationship. In it author Dr. Barbara Keesling offers practical knowledge and rare insight about lovemaking in a warm, encouraging tone. Drawing from years of professional experience, Keesling explores the profound, complex, and soulful powers of sexuality. She explains that sexual exchange between loving partners provides all the elements for a happy, healthy life: touch, intimacy, communication, physical activity, and playfulness.

256 pages ... 14 illus. ... Paperback ... $13.95 ... Available June 1998

SIMULTANEOUS ORGASM & Other Joys of Sexual Intimacy *by* Michael Riskin, Ph.D., and Anita Banker-Riskin, M.A.

For those of you who think "taking turns" is a fact of life, simultaneous orgasm can be liberating. It brings you into the moment and it focuses on the essence of your relationship and connection. For most couples, simultaneous orgasms happen accidentally, but with this book any couple can easily learn to enjoy them at will. Based on techniques developed at the Human Sexuality Institute, this book outlines an easy-to-follow, step-by-step program with specific techniques for partners to become orgasmic first separately, then simultaneously — to the point where they can experience every orgasm together.

240 pages ... 10 b&w photos ... Paperback $14.95 ... Hard cover $24.95

SUPER SENSUAL SEX: Awakening the Passion in Your Lover and Yourself *by* Beverly Engel

All of life is a sensual experience. While we live in a highly sexual culture, it is not very attuned to *sensual* pleasures. *Sensual Sex* shows readers that by becoming more attuned to their five senses they can develop an increasingly erotic relationship with their body and their partner's body. Offering a series of innovative touching and sensuality exercises, *Sensual Sex* helps couples reconnect with their bodies' exquisite pleasure, to drink in delicious sensations, and to luxuriate in each others senses.

256 pages … 10 b&w photos … Paperback $13.95 … Available October 1998

Prices subject to change

ORDER FORM

10% DISCOUNT on orders of $50 or more –
20% DISCOUNT on orders of $150 or more –
30% DISCOUNT on orders of $500 or more –
On cost of books for fully prepaid orders

NAME

ADDRESS

CITY/STATE ZIP/POSTCODE

PHONE COUNTRY

TITLE	QTY	PRICE	TOTAL
Treat Your Back Without Surgery		@ $14.95	
Menopause Without Medecine		@ $14.95	
Her Healthy Heart		@ $14.95	
Running on Empty		@ $14.95	
Please list other titles below:			
		@ $	
		@ $	
		@ $	
		@ $	
		@ $	
		@ $	

Shipping costs
First book: $3.00 by book post; $4.50 by UPS or to ship outside the U.S.
Each additional book: $1.00
For rush orders and bulk shipments call us at (800) 266-5592

SUBTOTAL ______
Less discount @ ______ % ( )
TOTAL COST OF BOOKS ______
Calif. residents add sales tax ______
Shipping & handling ______
TOTAL ENCLOSED ______
Please pay in U.S. funds only

❏ Check ❏ Money Order ❏ Visa ❏ M/C ❏ Discover

Card # ______________________ Exp date ______

Signature ______________________

Complete and mail to:

Hunter House Inc., Publishers
PO Box 2914, Alameda CA 94501-0914
Orders: 1-800-266-5592 . . . ordering@hunterhouse.com
Phone (510) 865-5282 Fax (510) 865-4295

❏ Check here to receive our FREE book catalog

TYB 3/98